Animal Hospital

Animal

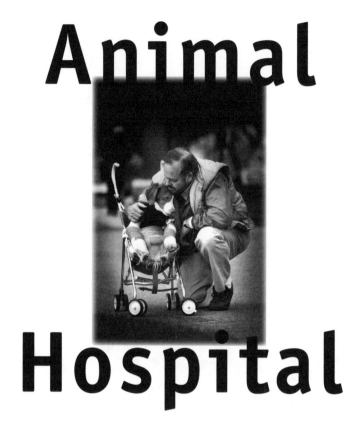

Hospital

STEPHEN SAWICKI

Chicago Review Press

Library of Congress Cataloging-in-Publication Data
Sawicki, Stephen.
      Animal hospital/Stephen Sawicki.
      227p. cm.
      ISBN 1-55652-274-6; paperback edition 1-55652-281-9
      1. Angell Memorial Animal Hospital (Jamaica Plain, Boston, Mass.)—
Anecdotes. 2. Veterinary hospitals—Massachusetts—Boston—Anecdotes. 3.
Veterinary medicine—Massachusetts—Boston—Anecdotes. 4. Veterinarians—
Massachusetts—Boston—Anecdotes. 5. Animals—Massachusetts—Boston—
Anecdotes. I. Title.
      SF604.62.M42A547 1996
      636.08'32'0974461—dc20   96–5732
                                        CIP

Cover photo: Yowser and his owner Don Ayles.
George Martell, courtesy *Boston Herald.*

© 1996 by Stephen Sawicki
All rights reserved
First paperback edition
Published by Chicago Review Press, Incorporated
814 North Franklin Street
Chicago, Illinois 60610
ISBN 1-55652-281-9
Printed in the United States of America
5 4 3 2 1

In memory of June Evelyn Sawicki

Contents

Preface   ix

Acknowledgments   xi

Introduction   1

P A R T   O N E   *Angells*

1. J.P.   7

2. Morris   11

3. Gamb   17

4. Rookie   27

5. Brum   35

6. Anthony   45

7. Carp   51

8. Decision   61

P A R T   T W O   *Inside*

9. Incoming   67

10. Waiting   75

11. Backshop   81

12. The Battle   89

P A R T   T H R E E   *Working*

13. Night   97

14. Dr. Feelgood   109

15. The Cutting Room   117

16. Vivos Docent   123

PART FOUR *Humaniacs*

17. Roots   135

18. Easter   149

19. Hunter   153

20. Hero   163

PART FIVE *Sanctuary*

21. Change   177

22. Fontaine   187

23. Challenge   199

24. Gone Fishing   203

25. Away   207

26. Abbey   211

Epilogue   223

Preface

THIS IS AN ACCOUNT OF MY YEAR INSIDE ANGELL
Memorial Animal Hospital in Boston, a world-renowned medical
center for pets.

Throughout my stay I made an effort to make sure that clients
and other visitors I observed were aware that I was a reporter. In some
instances, though emergencies in particular, such formalities were
impossible. Therefore, with privacy in mind, I have elected to use
pseudonyms for several clients and their pets. One veterinarian, who
is only mentioned briefly, is also given a fictional name.

Most of what follows is based on firsthand observation and
interviews. In some instances, particularly chapter 17, about the history of Angell Memorial and the Massachusetts Society for the
Prevention of Cruelty to Animals (MSPCA), I heavily relied on published material.

Among the MSPCA publications that were particularly helpful
were *Autobiographical Sketches and Personal Recollections*, by George T.
Angell, 1908; the monthly magazine *Our Dumb Animals*, 1868–1972,
which became *Animals,* 1972–present; *Fifty Years of the Angell Memorial
Animal Hospital,* by Gerry B. Schnelle, VMD, C. Lawrence Blakely,
VMD, and Gus W. Thornton, DVM, 1965; and *Three Decades of Angell
Memorial Animal Hospital,* by Gerry B. Schnelle, VMD, 1956.

Books I found useful included *The Animal Estate,* Harriet
Ritvo, Harvard University Press, 1987; *Men, Beasts, and Gods,* Gerald
Carson, Charles Scribner's Sons, 1972; *Reckoning with the Beast,* James
Turner, The Johns Hopkins University Press, 1980; and *The Woman
Who Wrote Black Beauty*, Susan Chitty, Hodder and Stoughton,
London, 1971.

This obviously is not a technical, scientific book, but I did spend a lot of time leafing through a variety of references and textbooks to better grasp what I was seeing. The ones I came back to time and again were *The Merck Veterinary Manual,* Seventh Edition, Merck & Co., 1991; *Small Animal Medical Diagnosis,* Michael D. Lorenz and Larry M. Cornelius, J. B. Lippincott, 1987; and *Veterinary Ethics,* Jerrold Tannenbaum, Williams & Wilkins, 1989.

Acknowledgments

IMAGINE HAVING A REPORTER COME TO YOUR WORK-
place and look over your shoulder—not just for an hour or a day or
even a week, but for one solid year. As someone who has strolled
along the beach while stacks of work sat undone, I must admit that
even I would not exactly embrace the concept. From the time that I
first suggested this project to the powers that be at the Massachusetts
Society for the Prevention of Cruelty to Animals (MSPCA), however, I have met with minimal resistance and a lot of kindness.

This project would never have gotten off the ground without
the friendly support of Marilyn McCunney in public relations and, in
turn, the approval of Gus Thornton, the MSPCA's president; Peter
Theran, vice president of health and hospitals; and Paul Gambardella,
chief of staff at Angell Memorial Animal Hospital. My gratitude to
each of them.

For my day-to-day work, I am in debt to my primary subjects
for their cooperation, understanding, and patience. Gambardella, I
know, defended this project to tentative staffers, to the point of telling
a group of wary interns that if they were in fact doing anything they
were afraid of people knowing about, well, they shouldn't be doing it
in the first place. Bless you, Paul.

Thanks, too, to James Carpenter, Lynne Morris, and Douglas
Brum, overworked people who shared with me prodigious amounts
of their time, feelings, experiences, and insights.

Like any reporter setting foot on a new landscape, I was always
seeking friendly faces for help and guidance at Angell. Sometimes,
too, I just needed to shoot the breeze. For making my load lighter and
for simply being kind souls, my special appreciation to Nancy
Crowley, Nancy Cuddyer, Joan Fontaine, Rose Henle, and Jennifer

Snow, as well as to Alesia Jillett and Arlyne Koopmann in the chief of staff's office.

Over the course of this book, my own dog was a full-fare patient at Angell. Thanks always to Jean Duddy, our veterinarian since puppyhood.

Any attempt to list the many other individuals at Angell and other branches of the MSPCA who contributed to this project would inevitably fall short. I am grateful, of course, to those who allowed me to observe as they went through their daily jobs. Many people were formally interviewed at length. Not a few helped in little ways every day that I set foot in the hospital. My appreciation to all concerned, and my regrets at being unable to thank you individually.

Angell's clients, of course, were also crucial to this book. I am indebted to innumerable pet owners, and their animals, for talking with me and letting me sit in on appointments. Thanks in particular to Anthony Bonacorso and Thomas Perkins and his family.

Far away from Angell my debts of gratitude are equally great. Thank you to Merritt Clifton, editor of the excellent monthly newspaper *Animal People,* for his insights into the world of non-profit organizations for animals. My appreciation also to Penny Holewa, archivist, Old Sturbridge Village; Kenneth C. Cramer, archivist, Dartmouth College Library; and Ken Gold.

Animal Hospital would not have come to be without the contributions, none small, of some good-hearted people. Leslie Graham, Mary Alice Welsh, Merri Kaye, Mary Beth Fox, Alan Greenstein, Jan Engle, and Janet Fillmore each made special efforts on behalf of me and this book that will long be remembered. Also, Jim Wood, a writer and friend from Shaker Heights, Ohio, was kind enough to evaluate an early draft of my manuscript. And photographer Steve Liss, who always has plenty to keep him busy, was more than generous with his time and talents. My thanks to all.

My family and friends were also there for me, as they always have been. They did a world of good by doing what friends do—listening, suggesting, and, at times, judiciously holding their tongues. From California to Ohio to New York, my love.

My thanks also to an old friend and many people's favorite teacher, Verne Edwards, for long keeping the faith. He also read and line-edited an early version of this manuscript, a chore that is much appreciated.

Cheers, too, to everyone at Chicago Review Press. Amy Teschner, former editorial director, and her successor Cynthia Sherry, in particular, are among my personal heroes.

In closing, it might seem a waste to express my gratitude to my dog, Abbey. She remains a nonreader, preferring twisted sticks, peculiar smells, and a luckless pursuit of seagulls along the ocean. No one and no thing, though, could have been better for my spirits over the long haul than the company of this peaceable animal.

Perhaps the man who used to do my taxes put it best one day when we were going over my finances, scavenging for additional deductions. In frustration, I jokingly asked whether we could somehow include the dog.

"Absolutely," he said, never looking up from his figures. "She's a consultant."

Absolutely.

For he shall give his angels charge over
thee to keep thee in all thy ways.
They shall bear thee up in their hands,
lest thou dash thy foot against a stone.

—PSALM 91:11–12, King James Version

Introduction

SEVERAL YEARS AGO, SHORTLY AFTER I BECAME THE owner of a golden retriever puppy, some friends suggested that I might find a good veterinarian at a place called Angell Memorial Animal Hospital.

I was fairly new to Boston and brand new to anything having to do with health care for a pet, yet I knew a little about Angell. Shortly after arriving in town, I had written a freelance article for *Animals,* a national magazine published by Angell's mother organization, the Massachusetts Society for the Prevention of Cruelty to Animals (MSPCA). After finishing the piece, the final word on flea control, I moved on to other publications and stories and, for the most part, forgot about the place.

Then one day, accompanied by my two-month-old puppy, who was in need of an examination and shots, I found myself sitting in Angell's waiting room. Abbey was wide-eyed at every new person and pet that ambled by. I was dumbstruck myself at what I had stumbled upon.

Here was a hospital for animals that was big enough for people. A cardiologist was on staff. A neurologist. A gastroenterologist. A handful of surgeons. Interns, for heaven's sake. Residents. I looked around the waiting room and witnessed such a variety of pets and illnesses—not to mention the owners, who seemed so devoted. I came away feeling as if I had discovered some kind of *ER* for animals.

Over time, I would learn that veterinary medicine had grown up while I wasn't watching—and was still blossoming. Americans own as many as fifty-seven million dogs, sixty-seven million cats, and some thirty-five million exotics, from parrots to gerbils to lizards, according to one study. The 1995 American Animal Hospital Association Report—A Study of the Companion Animal Veterinary Services Market—found that in 1994 Americans spent $20 billion on their pets, with $8.5 billion going to veterinary care. These numbers are certain to rise, given another truth discovered by the American Animal Hospital Association survey: for whatever reason, more and more people have taken to humanizing their pets, dressing them in clothes, for example, and even leaving them messages on the answering machine. Of the pet owners surveyed, 70 percent considered their pets like children, and 54 percent admitted to being emotionally dependent on them.

There sat Angell, right on the front lines of the pet revolution in animal health, rivaled only by New York's Animal Medical Center and some of the better veterinary schools, with one of the heaviest caseloads, and doing everything from routine care to hip replacements and brain surgery.

Over the months after my first visit, I often wondered about the hospital. The medicine was intriguing, to be sure. But the people who worked there were what I kept thinking about. How was it that their lives brought them to such a place, performing such work? What was the nature of their daily lives? What did they see and feel and think? What stories of tragedy and triumph had they been keeping to themselves all these years?

Finally, I contacted the MSPCA to feel them out about a book idea that had evolved in my mind. In essence, I wanted a year's access to the hospital, to look over the shoulders of its staff. During the next few months, I would meet with Marilyn McCunney, then the society's director of public relations; Peter Theran, the society's vice president of health and hospitals; and Paul Gambardella, Angell's chief of staff.

The officers and staff were used to media attention. Angell was known worldwide. (In Tokyo, in fact, an independent veterinary center was named after it—Angell Memorial Hiroo Central Hospital, which opened in 1992.) In the Boston hospital's heyday in the fifties and sixties, celebrities from around the country brought their pets in. Elvis Presley's sick chow chow, flown into town from Memphis, was perhaps the most famous patient. While these days most patients are from New England, some people—such as California-based actress Loretta Swit—have been known to fly their pets long distances for treatment at Angell.

Television and film crews, magazine writers, and newspaper reporters were always filtering in and out during my stay. A team from "Rescue 911" spent a few days with the staff. "This hospital is in a fishbowl," Paul Gambardella told me almost proudly. "Everybody sees through our walls and is watching us swim."

And so, I spent a year watching the Angell fish swim.

Gambardella proved to be an ardent supporter of my project. He allowed me almost unlimited run of the hospital and said no to surprisingly few requests. Certain personnel meetings, for example, were closed to me, but not much else.

My goal was to tell Angell's story through its people. Within a couple months, I found five or six with whom I would spend most of my time. Did they typify Angell? I think they did. However, I spent less time than I would have liked with certain other immensely talented veterinarians and staffers. Some were too busy or disinclined to deal with a writer at their heels. Cardiologist Neil Harpster, beloved by hordes of clients and invaluable to his bosses, was kind enough when I approached him, but he simply ran at speeds that made him less than the perfect subject.

Which is not to say that the others made it easy. Lynne Morris initially resisted having me around but, like any self-respecting intern, acquiesced when I brought a free pizza into the equation. Staff veterinarian Douglas Brum, meanwhile, always seemed to be caught in an internal struggle between his typical race-walker pace and a speed slow enough to be polite to me. Pathologist James Carpenter was a fervent champion of punctuality; though he uttered no complaint, I always felt deep shame on those occasions when he happened to see me slink in late for a lecture or meeting.

At times some would have preferred that I not be around at all.

One day when I was shadowing Gambardella, he spun around and pointed at me. "You! Just stay here! I'm going to the bathroom!" Another time he mused to his assistant that he would be able to get some paperwork done as soon as I "metastasized."

On the days when Angell was slow, I would sit by the vending machines, where I could watch people passing by, read the newspaper, and wait for visitors. Kathy Anderson, a kindly woman from the financial office, who has since died, liked to tell me about the mysteries she was reading. Intern Christopher Wong spoke of comic-book collecting. Longtime veterinarian Michael Bernstein filled me with hospital lore and urged me down the hall to meet his favorite clients. And everyone had tidbits—gossip, funny stories, and gripes.

One wild-mannered veterinarian—not one of my main subjects—was notorious for making obnoxious comments to people around the hospital, insults that were too outrageous to repeat or ever take seriously. The remarks were the stuff of shock-jock radio—a call for attention, I guessed—as he desecrated everything from a person's sexual proclivities to their questionable parentage. He never did it to outsiders, though; it was more of a familial thing.

One day I was in a hallway chatting with someone when he ambled by. "Don't talk to that delinquent bastard!" he shouted, referring to me.

Thank you, I should have said.

I was in.

PART ONE *Angells*

Hear ye not the hum of mighty workings?

—JOHN KEATS, "Sonnet XIV"

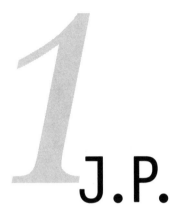

J.P.

THE ANGELL MEMORIAL ANIMAL HOSPITAL IS LOCATED in the Boston neighborhood of Jamaica Plain. To get there each day, I would ride the Green Line train from Brighton to the Brookline Village stop, then walk the remaining mile.

Mine was a route dominated by the automobile, many of which tore by fast enough to keep me ever alert against sudden vehicular death. Each day the narrow Jamaicaway thoroughfare, which ran parallel to my path, carried thousands of commuters maniacally charging in and out of the city, heedless of pedestrians and other terrain dwellers.

Other forces of darkness were apparently lurking. On the sparsely wooded path I followed, the sidewalk doubling as a bicycle route, someone had spray-painted a warning: "MUGGERS AHEAD—DANGER." I was never waylaid, but someone must have been. The very presence of such an admonition underscored the fact that the turf was changing. This was where privileged Brookline met hardscrabble Jamaica Plain. Though anyone could have scrawled the message, my guess is that it was one of the young professionals or spandex-clad bicyclists who followed this path to their apartments or the subway and wanted their fellow man to learn from their sad experience.

For me it was a pleasant walk. My path led past a scenic pond and a well-tended park, complete with a baseball diamond and a field where dog owners took their animals for romps. A bit past the ballfield, I warily crossed Jamaicaway and hiked up a steep residential street, lined with double-decker homes, toward South Huntington Avenue and my destination.

Every day about halfway up the hill, I would be struck by the tremendous brick structure that loomed like a giant rising sun. Surrounding the expansive five-story building—encompassing one entire city block—was an eight-foot-high brick wall topped by rusty barbed wire. It all looked like an ancient penitentiary or an asylum from the darker days of treating mental illness. It intimidated. And it owned the horizon.

This was The Angell.

Some days, rather than go straight into the fortress, where I spent my days watching veterinarians attempting to heal animals, I followed the brick wall around back and surveyed the neighborhood, seeking to learn what was being so fiercely guarded against. As it turned out, it was the neighborhood itself: Jamaica Plain, or, as the locals called it, J.P.

Like with most urban neighborhoods, the decades had washed across Jamaica Plain, transforming it. In the nineteenth century, the area provided an escape for the well-to-do, who retreated here to summer homes. Notorious Boston mayor James Michael Curley owned a handsome Georgian revival mansion in Jamaica Plain. Helen Keller attended the nation's first kindergarten for the blind where the animal hospital today sits.

Nowadays Jamaica Plain is increasingly low rent. Community optimists like to point to the neighborhood's mix of Hispanics, African Americans, Asians, Irish Americans, and all the rest as proof positive that varied races and cultures can live and work together. Indeed, many people love the neighborhood and proudly call it home. Yet for all the talk of racial harmony, it is also true that many of J.P.'s residents simply can afford little else. Wedged between Brookline and Boston's tough Roxbury neighborhood, J.P. is a hybrid, its populace a mix of hard-core poor, blue-collar laborers, low-paid professionals, and students.

If you read the Boston newspapers, you know about the periodic slayings that take place in lonely J.P. apartments or the real-life shoot-'em-ups that erupt every now and then in the streets. You know enough that if you are out walking at night, you bring a friend. Or a dog. The larger the better, whatever the species.

Still, the streets and sidewalks that front Angell are not particularly threatening. The hospital is just up the road from the modern glimmer of the Veterans Administration Medical Center and an assortment of smaller health and social service organizations. Across the street are some apartment buildings. Trolley tracks still run down the center of South Huntington, though they have been unused for years.

City buses, meanwhile, rumble past the animal hospital. Police cruisers scream by. Mostly, though, it is endless car and truck traffic streaming into or out of the city, with every third or fourth vehicle in need of muffler work.

Behind Angell Memorial, where the fortress kisses the heart of the neighborhood, one treads more carefully. The wall back there was covered with graffiti: "VIVA LA LUCHA HEROICA DE LAS MASAS HAITIANAS!" read one message. "HOW MANY DEAD!" said another. Other markings were apolitical, the signature scrawlings of assorted vandals and hoodlums. Eventually, the graffiti would become so pervasive and unsightly that the city of Boston would lean on Angell's mother organization, the MSPCA, about cleaning it, since the wall was its property.

Out back are residences. Some neighbors take obvious pride in their property and surroundings. Other structures, though, are dilapidated and getting worse, marring the landscape.

A block away is J.P.'s central business district, home of discount shops and diners. Hack and Slash Glass and Aluminum is here, as is the Centre Boutique, where a sign in the window promises "Good prices in bad times."

All is abustle. The traffic. The mothers loading and unloading screaming babies from cars. In the summer shirtless men cluster on the corners. It isn't hard to find someone hustling change—if not worse.

All of this is in strange contrast to the garrison that houses Angell Memorial and the MSPCA. Inside is another world. The grounds, including the parking lots, are spacious. A bronze sculpture of a horse, a tribute to the hospital's original patients, rears before the building. The lawn is lush. Well tended shrubbery and flowers are all over. All with nary a view of the mean streets outside.

One of the staffers told me of an old-timer from the neighborhood who over the years periodically made his way into the fortress, up the concrete ramp that led to the automatic sliding doors, and into Angell's waiting room—sans pet. There he sat and whiled away the hours reading his newspaper, speaking to no one, bothering no one. I smiled at the very idea.

Eventually, I thought I understood. Of course, tranquillity was not to be found here, amidst the cries of ailing cats, the barks of impatient dogs, and the tedious chitchat of their owners.

Perhaps peace and quiet were not what he sought, however. Perhaps it was sanctuary.

2 Morris

IT WAS MIDMORNING THE DAY AFTER THE SUPER Bowl, when Matteo, a one-hundred-pound rottweiler, came into Angell wrapped in the muscular arms of his owner.

Anthony Bonacorso had awakened that day to find his dog, just a year and a half old, at death's door, vomiting and urinating over and over. When Bonacorso helped him to his feet, the dog wobbled around the house like a drunkard, barely able to keep his balance. It was, to say the least, unusual.

Matteo, named after one of Anthony's cousins in Italy, was a "rotty" through and through. Sleekly black, with rust coloring to his muzzle and chest, the dog displayed such musculature that one wondered whether he and his weight lifter owner pumped the iron together.

If not that, they certainly shared plenty of other activities. Drives. Hikes. Family outings. Anthony even brought Matteo to parties, where Bonacorso's friends greeted Matteo like one of the gang. Just the day before, in fact, Matteo had joined Bonacorso at a Super Bowl get-together with some buddies.

Bonacorso, who was twenty-six and taking business classes at Boston College, searched his mind that next Monday morning for what the dog could have gotten into. Seemingly from nowhere he heard himself say, "Antifreeze."

Sunday's Super Bowl gathering had been at a construction company that Anthony owned just north of the city, not far from his home. The weather had been frigid. To prevent the building's pipes from freezing, the plumber had come by a few days earlier and poured antifreeze in the toilet. While the party was going on around the big-screen television in the offices upstairs, Bonacorso's dog somehow found his way to the bathroom and began slurping from the john.

Bonacorso had no idea what had occurred, and he failed to pay much heed despite noticing that the dog had a touch of diarrhea and had relieved himself on the rug. Also, when he put Matteo down in the building's garage for a while, the animal uncharacteristically kept urinating all over the place.

It was not until the next morning around eight o'clock that Anthony realized something was seriously wrong. He had just awoken and saw Matteo stretched out in the living room. "Normally, what I would do to keep the dog on guard, I would play little games with him," related Bonacorso. "I would sneak up on him all the time while he was sleeping and scare him, grab his leg or whatever. It was a game. Sometimes I would catch him; sometimes he would catch me sneaking up on him."

This time, though, Anthony met no resistance, just a nod of recognition. When he set his hand where the dog's muzzle had been, he discovered that the floor was soaked. Matteo was lying in his own urine.

Anthony tried to help the dog up, but the animal was so weak, he could barely stand. He swayed back and forth. Matteo's rear legs seemed to have atrophied overnight. Drool hung from his mouth in ropes.

"I don't know why," Anthony recalled, "I just thought 'antifreeze.' I felt God was giving me a message. I immediately picked him up, put him in the Jeep, and drove here like an animal. I *flew* here. I ran more red lights than any day in my life."

Intern Lynne Morris was on emergencies, or as they call it at Angell, "walk-in duty," when Matteo arrived. Morris, in her mid-twenties, looked the part of a young veterinarian. She wore her long, light-brown hair pulled behind her head and braided down the back of her doctor's coat. A battered, orange-covered formulary was ever-present in the side pocket. Underneath was a casual button-down shirt. And like everyone under age forty at Angell, she preferred comfortable athletic shoes—in Morris's case, white leather Reeboks—over anything dressier.

Morris's classical features and passive expression sometimes made it hard to gauge her mood. At times her work made her cry, and other times it stirred her anger, but she tended to present a patient, calm expression, a mirror of her general disposition.

Morris looked Matteo over. She pressed her stethoscope to his side. She tossed out some routine questions for Anthony, who told her that if the dog had drunk antifreeze, it was probably twelve to fifteen hours earlier. It was anyone's guess how much he had consumed.

From everything she saw and all that Bonacorso told her, Morris said, it was a good bet that the dog had indeed ingested antifreeze, which, with ethylene glycol as its main component, was deadly to man or beast.

Less certain was the dog's chance for survival. When ethylene glycol is in the system too long—more than twelve hours—the odds of saving an animal are diminished. The liver will already have metabolized the chemical into a toxin. The kidneys, in particular, can then become severely damaged and rendered incapable of producing urine. With toxins running rampant through its system, an animal often suffers—truly suffers—a slow, awful death.

Bonacorso told Morris that money was no object, that she and her fellow doctors should do whatever was necessary. Emotional clients tend to make such remarks. Morris knew that as often as not, money was a problem. Overwrought owners are simply in no mind-frame to admit it.

Bonacorso, though, truly could put his hands on whatever it would cost—perhaps as much as eleven thousand dollars—to throw everything the hospital could at saving Matteo. Bonacorso was not rich, but he was willing to spend what he had if Matteo had a chance. "Just imagine if you had all the money in the world," he would later say, "but a broken heart."

So it began. Matteo was taken into the intensive care unit. There he was given intravenous 4-methylpyrazole, a relatively new and expensive drug, which, if given soon enough, could prevent the toxin from taking effect.

He also had an ultrasound biopsy. An image was taken of the dog's innards on the ultrasound machine. Then a needle was inserted into one of the kidneys, and bits of tissue were pulled out to be examined down in pathology. This would reveal the severity of the damage.

By the next day, Morris saw that the dog was not improving. Among other signs, blood tests showed his creatinine—a by-product of muscle breakdown that is usually eliminated by the kidneys—still at a high level. Matteo had not urinated in almost twenty-four hours.

Morris and Alicia Faggella, who headed intensive care, talked with Bonacorso about dialysis. It was not something that was done often, but if he wanted, they could try. The alternative was almost certain death.

That afternoon Matteo was wheeled into surgery, anesthetized, and his belly opened. A peritoneal dialysis catheter, with a tube leading out from the dog, was placed inside the abdominal cavity, alongside the liver, kidney, and intestines. For the next few weeks, if need be, fluids would be infused into the dog's abdomen, drawing the toxins from the blood and, with the help of the dialysis catheter, out of his system.

It was, in essence, like installing a primitive kidney to rid the body of the toxins. It was not as efficient as the dialysis machines used in human hospitals, but it still had the potential to save the day.

Soon telephone calls began pouring into the hospital. The people who worked in the liaison office, who served as links between the veterinarians and their patients, shook their heads in disbelief. Friends of Bonacorso were calling every ten minutes for updates. "Hi!" they would say. "I'm a friend of Matteo's. How's he doing?"

Anthony himself went on a binge of learning whatever he could about kidneys and treatment for a problem of this sort. He also raised some eyebrows when he asked whether, if worse came to worst, the doctors could possibly retain some of his dog's sperm for breeding. He put this question to Betsy Allen, a liaison. She came back with the response from one of the doctors that it was out of the question, that even if the sperm were unaffected by the toxins, the hospital lacked facilities for freezing it.

In her ten years at the hospital, Allen had grown accustomed to requests of all kinds. She had seen, for instance, owners who appeared with the bodies of their pets, mangled by automobiles, and asked that after everything else, did Betsy think they could clip the nails? Once, to placate an elderly man, she conducted an impromptu funeral service for his dog. Now someone wanted sperm. Such requests sounded bizarre, but Betsy knew they were simply the sounds of people trying to cope.

Still, Allen could not help smiling as she headed back toward the liaison office: she herself was about to undergo artificial insemination. She later suggested that, after denying Anthony's request, "I *should* have added, 'But perhaps, sir, we could have a sample from you.'"

3
Gamb

PAUL GAMBARDELLA STEPPED INTO DIRTY SURGERY and sensed that something was awry. With the weekend but a few hours away, the chief of staff expected to at least hear the chatter of the surgical technicians and orderlies as they looked forward to two days off. Instead, the room was hushed.

Usually this area of Angell Memorial Animal Hospital was bustling. "Dirty" only in that it was not sterile, this was where medical interns and staff doctors brought their patients for cast changes, treatment of skin wounds, and any number of low-risk surgical procedures. Often the place had the air of a bus depot, with rackety gurneys rolling in and out and busy people coming and going.

On this Friday in January, though only a few employees were hard at it. Everyone else—seven or eight people in all, most in sky blue scrubs—had paused to watch a drama unfold at one of the stainless steel treatment tables. Some of the spectators bent over the silvery tabletops. Others leaned against entranceways. The rest stood to the side, arms folded, intrigued.

The focus of their attention was Nora, a three-year-old

German shepherd–husky mix, and one of the residents, Debbie Slayton.

Nora had not been urinating. When the dog had come into the hospital as an emergency two days earlier, Lynne Morris suspected that something, a tumor perhaps, was pressing against the dog's ure-thra, causing the blockage. It turned out to be a perianal abscess.

The dog was now anesthetized and stretched out in the least enviable of positions. Chest down, her snout was pointed to the pale yellow, cinder block wall. And her hindquarters, tail tied off to the side, were on display for any and all viewers.

Slayton had sliced a three-inch incision alongside the dog's anus to clear out whatever pus or other matter had gathered deep within. To her surprise, she found remnants of a previous operation: black-ened, bloody gobs of a surgical packing material with the consisten-cy of rice pudding. Although dissolvable, the stuff had yet to fully break down and disappear. Dutifully, Slayton set about removing it.

Minutes later, when her work was almost done, it happened. Deep in the surgical cavity where a network of vessels met, a weak-ened wall gave way, and blood began to flow. "It was like Niagara Falls coming toward me," Slayton later recalled.

Similar events happen often in surgery, veterinary or otherwise. For the doctor, the first and most important step is to remain calm. Most surgeons will simply take a deep breath, probe around for the damaged vessel, and seal it off as soon as possible. With smaller ani-mals, time can be precious. With a big dog like Nora, some delay can be tolerated—some.

Slayton looked into the opening, which was finger-length deep. Space was tight, two or three inches across, and with the blood pour-ing forth, pinpointing the new injury site was difficult. She inserted her shiny, scissor-shaped hemostat, attempting to clamp off the ves-sels. Time and again she just missed.

On the wall clock overhead, a minute passed. Then a few more. Then some more. Blood coated Slayton's latex gloves. A crimson pud-dle formed on the floor. Several more near-misses.

Finally, with the blood loss mounting, the resident had a

strained, nervous look. She ordered that the equipment be set up for a blood transfusion. Eyes got big all around the room. To help her see, Slayton grabbed a suction tube, drawing blood away from the wound and into a rapidly filling glass container to her right.

Such was the scene that Paul Gambardella discovered this afternoon. Dressed in scrubs himself, he was already in the midst of a busy day. Work had started at seven-thirty with a seminar and took Gambardella headlong into a steady stream of veterinary and administrative duties. For Gambardella the orthopedic surgeon, the morning brought a two-hour pelvic operation on a dog named Rascal. For Gambardella the chief of staff, the afternoon held the unfinished paperwork for a new ultrasound machine and the need to investigate client complaints.

Gambardella's title excluded him from the racier conversations around the sprawling hospital. Any high jinx usually fell to a simmer when he entered a room. All the same, no one truly feared him. He was not a wholly intimidating presence. Had Gambardella been born canine, he would have been a Boston terrier, smallish but big enough to make you stiffen when he barked. At forty-five, he kept his weight steady at one hundred fifty pounds, the result of dietary habits that included no breakfast, just peanut butter cookies and a diet soft drink for lunch, then dinner.

His face, distinctly Italian, was pleasant. It was divided into thirds by his dark mustache, his thick eyebrows, and a thatch of hair in the center of his balding pate just above the forehead.

More telling than his appearance, though, was his approachable manner. Gambardella certainly had moments when his brown eyes flared. But Angell staffers knew well that he was more likely to subdue them with a yarn of one sort or another than to scream and stomp around. His humor leaned toward the corny. When someone mentioned ICU in conversation one day, Gambardella retorted, "I see you, too." Another time, after being informed of who was going to be acting hospital supervisor for the afternoon, he asked, "Who's she gonna be acting *like*?"

Now he stepped behind the resident and surveyed the bloody

pit with the matter-of-factness of a man sizing up new radials for the station wagon. "Need an extra pair of hands, Debbie?" he offered.

Slayton, concentrating on her work, said nothing. Gambardella watched for a bit. Then he walked over to a rack of supplies, opened a package of surgical gloves, and stretched them on. He was already on his way back when Slayton asked, "Uh, Paul, would you mind putting on some gloves?"

Crouching beside her, he gazed into the wound. Gambardella, too, made an attempt or two with the hemostat but failed. Then he put a finger deep inside, pressing it against the vessels to stem the red tide for a moment.

An orderly hurried over and adjusted a light directly behind the doctors' heads, to help illuminate the opening.

"You know," Gambardella said, "this reminds me of this cartoon I saw one time."

"It *does*?" Slayton replied. "This sure doesn't feel like a cartoon."

Gambardella ignored her. "There's this little boy with his finger in the dike—well, I'll tell you about it later."

Turning to the hemorrhaging dog, Gambardella looked, tried again with the hemostat, and stopped. He rubbed the back of his balding head, then his neck. "Geez," he said animatedly, "with this light I feel like I'm getting a sunburn here." Faces around the room grinned in spite of themselves. It was vintage Paul Gambardella.

Something less obvious came across as well: gone was the urgency of the moment. It was obvious that Gambardella wasn't worried. What for a few minutes had been the momentous question of *whether* the dog would be saved had now merely become a matter of *when*. And at this rate it probably would be after a quip or two more from the chief of staff.

Sure enough, Gambardella did manage to close down the flow, and the vessels were clipped shut. He turned to Slayton. "Anyway, I remember seeing this cartoon," he said. "There's a little boy, and he's got his finger in the dike. And in front of him there's this naked woman lying there, inviting him. But he can't reach her. And he's wrestling with himself over whether he should save the city or be with this woman." Gambardella laughed out loud. "That's what this made me think of."

It also reminded him of a case he had seen years before, when he was a surgery resident at the University of Minnesota. A fellow doctor, Gambardella said, while repairing the pelvis of a tiny dog, was drilling through the bone and accidentally pierced a sizable vessel underneath. Between the smallness of the animal and the pelvis obscuring the new injury, the doctor could not act fast enough. The dog rapidly bled to death. It is rare to see it, Gambardella said, yet it does happen.

But not today. "Thank you, Paul," Slayton said as Gambardella headed out.

"Oh, no problem."

He ran his hand over the back of his skull, lingering on his bald spot, as he neared the exit. "Boy," he muttered to himself, "that *light* . . ."

WHEN PAUL GAMBARDELLA WAS A BOY, THE LAST PLACE he wanted to spend his summers was his father's veterinary clinic. He preferred being out playing with his buddies. But when Paul was thirteen or fourteen years old, in the early sixties, John Gambardella enlisted him as a kennel boy. There he would serve, for about forty dollars a week, until graduating from high school.

Paul, the eldest of three boys and four girls, did a bit of everything around the practice. He cleaned cages, answered the phone, and took care of whatever else his father needed. As time went on, Paul was trusted to perform fecal examinations and assist in surgery, furnishing this instrument or that one while his father labored with a troublesome fracture.

Although the elder Gambardella had a number of associates over the years, his practice in Branford, Connecticut, outside of New Haven, was largely a one-man show. In the days before specialists, he covered the gamut of veterinary services, from exams to shots to surgery. He even did some grooming. What's more, he kept up with the latest techniques. Sometimes he would even push up the highway to attend training seminars at Boston's renowned Angell Memorial Animal Hospital.

Paul could not help but ingest tremendous amounts of information, from how to speak to clients to how to hold a scalpel. Paul saw his father perform bone pinnings, for example, when most vets were relying on splints. Paul fainted during surgery once, but he blamed that on an empty stomach, the hot lights, and the tedium of assisting. Whatever the case, that rite of passage for many a young veterinarian was out of the way early, and Paul never hit the floor again.

Among Paul's jobs for his father was bathing and grooming several pets a day. He was fourteen or fifteen, old enough, his father believed, to perform the task as well as handle the responsibility. "Well, my dad had this grooming table," Gambardella recalled. "It was a three-sided table up against the wall, with a brace sticking out from the wall and a ring where you tied the animal, with a noose, to hold the animal there.

"The irresponsible teenager that I was at the time, I walked away from the dog I was working on to do something. I don't know what it was, but I left this dog alone on this table tied to this ring. And the dog jumped off the table and hung himself."

He paused. "And it died. That devastated me, I'll tell you. I never forgot it. That's the only time that I can recall making a mistake that directly related to the death of an animal."

Gambardella attended Saint Anselm College in New Hampshire, where he debated going on to dentistry school or medical school. Paul wanted to break from what his father did, to cut his own path. Around his junior year, though, he got to thinking that what he really loved was working with the animals. It began to seem silly not to pursue veterinary medicine just because it was also his father's line of work.

In general, veterinary school, like medical school and dental school, called for applicants to have fulfilled its particular entrance requirements but not necessarily to hold a bachelor's degree. Gambardella was never one to wait. He was accepted at the University of Pennsylvania and left St. Anselm after his junior year.

That summer he married his hometown girlfriend, Susie. (He bought her engagement ring with money saved from his summers working for his father.) They moved to Philadelphia and for four years lived close to the bone, dividing their worries between the cutthroats in Paul's classes and those who prowled the inner-city streets. In the end Paul came away with the award for the best clinic work as a senior and won an internship at the University of Minnesota.

It was during his internship that Paul turned the old surgery adage "See one, do one, teach one" on its ear. He was asked to instruct a class of veterinary students in spaying by actually performing the operation in front of them. "I didn't have the nerve to say I never spayed a dog," he remembered. "I had done some abdominal surgery. I figured taking the ovaries out really wasn't any different than taking the spleen out, so I said sure." When it was over, no one was the wiser.

Gambardella would spend two additional years in Minnesota as a surgery resident when specialization in the field was just taking hold. In what spare time he had, he also earned a master's degree in veterinary surgery.

He came to Angell in 1975 as a staff surgeon, one of the rare hires in those days not to have been an Angell intern. What's more, he was the hospital's first board-certified surgeon to have undergone a full-blown residency.

Gambardella needed about ten years before he felt completely comfortable in surgery. Over time, complications became rare. Now it hardly mattered what kind of orthopedic surgery—from mending a shattered limb to performing a total hip replacement—was needed. Almost every new case became a variation of something that had already lain prostrate before him. Angell's heavy caseload gave him such an assortment of injuries to repair that even the most complicated bone surgery drew hardly a pause.

Like his counterparts in the human field, Gambardella regarded his work in terms of creation, as an art. Yet he spoke of surgery like a craftsman. "It's no different than building a deck," he told me one day, "or putting together a model airplane. You've actually done something. You've opened up an animal and removed the tumor and closed him back up. You've opened up the leg and put it back together, and now the animal can walk again. It's a production, and it's a challenging product to make."

He had been chief of staff at Angell Memorial—a title that by itself ranked him among the heavyweights in veterinary medicine—for three years. To many veterinarians, such a position would be the crown of their careers. Gambardella, however, said he never longed for the job. He had left Angell's employ once, though not the building, to teach small-animal surgery for the fledgling veterinary school at Tufts University, which for several years shared Angell's facilities. When Tufts eventually opened its own hospital, Paul chose to return to Angell.

What landed him in the chief of staff job was a shake-up at the top of the MSPCA, which was struggling with massive financial woes. One president was pressured to resign; Angell's chief of staff then, Gus Thornton, ascended to the throne. Gambardella was suddenly elevated to top man at the hospital, at first on a temporary basis, then permanently.

But the chief of staff position was being redefined. Previous chiefs of staff were veterinary men through and through. Though they had dealt with administrative matters and budgets, these were nothing like the duties expected of Gambardella. From on high came strict budget requirements and a demand that Gambardella eliminate $650,000 in spending from Angell's $8 million budget in one year. Budget cutting became the order of the day, year after year. Paul was ordered to develop new programs, find new revenue sources, and cut expenses.

Gambardella also inherited internal dissension and, in the end, fired a popular, longtime department head. This led to a sex discrimination lawsuit, with several years of legal wrangling before it would go to court.

Thirty miles away in North Grafton, meanwhile, Tufts had opened its own not-for-profit, specialty animal hospital, and Angell was beginning to feel the pinch. New private practices, including specialty practices, were springing up around Greater Boston. The trend promised to continue, especially with Tufts churning out local talent annually.

Sometimes all of it began to eat at Gambardella. On bad days he drove home to suburban Medfield wondering what he was doing in this job, when all he wanted was to be a surgeon. "There are a lot of times when I say I don't want to do this," he said. "I'm not made for this. I should be down on the assembly line with nobody bothering me."

Therein was Gambardella's dilemma. The demands of the chief of staff job increasingly kept him out of surgery. His salary was now better than $120,000; while private practice might have been more lucrative, Gambardella was doing significantly better than he did on Angell's "assembly line." The money would help put three boys through college. One was already a freshman at the University of Maine, while the others—a high schooler and a sixth-grader—were not far behind.

Despite the many pulls on his time, Paul attended surgery rounds every morning at eight o'clock sharp. He kept up his journal reading. However, he could see appointments only a couple mornings or afternoons a week, and his hands were on a scalpel far less than he needed for complete satisfaction.

Sometimes Gambardella's spirits sagged. If he had no patients of his own, he would call down to surgery: "Need any help? I can even do some spays." And when surgery did summon him, Paul would toss his papers onto his desk and head downstairs as if his trolley were pulling out. "Gotta go," he would tell his administrative assistant. "They *need* me."

The other cutters all saw the melancholy in Paul's eyes. "He sits down by the window in surgery, and he howls," said one, James Boulay.

One day as Gambardella was finishing suturing a scruffy dog named Carlos, from whom he had just removed a tumor for a biopsy, a happy look spread across the man's Italian features. "Well, I'm looking forward to tomorrow," he said. "I'll be back in surgery. I hate that office. Those are problems that I can't solve. Down here I know the answers."

4
Rookie

THE OTHER INTERNS QUICKLY CAUGHT WIND OF Lynne Morris's case. Antifreeze-damaged dogs and cats were common at Angell, but to have someone willing to try dialysis was rare. Matteo was a case from which everyone could learn.

"Cool!" the interns said as they looked in on the gloomy rottweiler in intensive care. "Great case!" they told Morris when they saw her in the Hole, the cramped intern quarters on the first floor, or passed her in the hallways.

Lynne smiled, but the remarks were starting to annoy her. Here was a once-robust dog who was in trouble, and as every day passed he got deeper in it. Here was also a young man who was going to have to pay thousands of dollars and probably never see his dog walk out of here. Not much of it sounded great to her. "Everyone keeps telling me, 'Great case, great case,'" she said privately. "I don't *care* if it's a great case. I don't care about great cases. I just want them to get better."

Lynne's intern class consisted of nine women and three men. They came from all over the country, with a range of experiences and personalities. One intern had played professional tennis. Another worked for a while in the fashion industry. Still another had been heavily involved with marine mammals. There were those who had strong research backgrounds. Others had an animal-rights bent.

They also had much in common. All were white, with the exception of one woman of Asian descent. Most were in their mid-to-late twenties. All, of course, had known the rigors of veterinary school.

And most, at some point, had told curious strangers that they chose to be veterinarians rather than physicians because, frankly, they liked animals better than people. This kind of talk was, of course, just a way of making conversation. After all, as one staff doctor said, it was not often that Happy showed up at Angell by his lonesome, with a list of ailments and a Mastercard in his mouth. Working with animals would be the easiest part of the interns' jobs. Those who had trouble getting along with owners would find their stay at Angell torturous.

As it was, winter itself was grueling enough for interns at Angell. When they started in June, every day was new and thrilling. Each case, no matter how routine, was an education. For nearly six months, the learning curve climbed like an arrow shot straight into the sky. Come winter, and most of the newly minted veterinarians took on a faded look. Their learning had continued, but at a significantly diminished rate.

Now, long hours at the hospital showed on the interns' faces. They arrived before first light and left in the evening, rarely seeing much more than a glimpse of sunlight. Angell itself began to feel like once-favorite clothes worn far too often. Certain clients, once considered challenging, became full-scale burdens. Certain staff doctors who once bowed to the interns' newness to Angell, now set aside niceties. As each week passed, the interns knew that all of the staff doctors were privately evaluating their personalities, abilities, and trustworthiness. Some felt hated; none felt beloved.

In June all the interns had started fairly even. After they learned the paperwork, Angell protocols, and where everything was located, the class began to settle out. Some would never get very good at this work. Others, within a few months, showed an obvious knack.

Morris was a favorite of both the staff and clients. She worked hard, deciding early on to throw heart, soul, and most waking hours into the internship. Her fiancé, a physician, was in the Navy. She placed her two dogs in the care of her parents in the south-of-Boston suburb of Avon. For thirteen months and less than $15,000 in salary, Lynne signed her life over to chief of staff Paul Gambardella and his minions.

A willingness to labor long and hard ranked high in the minds of staff doctors when taking the measure of an intern. Morris tossed in a friendly nature as well. She even took a liking to some of the senior veterinarians feared by most interns.

Lynne disarmed owners—and irritated a few—by addressing them as if they were their pets' parents. The men were "dads," the women "moms." All cats, geriatrics included, were "kitties." Even the fiercest looking male dog she pronounced, with a pat, to be a "good boy."

Morris and her dozen fellow interns had recently passed the midway point of their program. Angell's internship, the first in the country when it started in the forties, was the most challenging of any in veterinary medicine. In terms of long hours and stress, it could also match anything human medicine threw at its youngest doctors.

Physicians, though, were required to serve internships; veterinarians were not. If this was "Ange-hell," as some called the place, it was a hell of their own choosing.

Unlike programs at similar-sized veterinary institutions, Angell outright gave its interns the power—and burden—of making the treatment decisions on their own cases. Help was available from the permanent staff, and the interns were told to seek it out. As an extra precaution, the older doctors also kept abreast of the interns' cases during rounds and at various other points in their days.

Unlike with most programs, no team of doctors or senior doctor worked up the intern's cases for them. At Angell, every intern learned the hardest part of being a veterinarian: living and dying with your own decisions—and having your patients do the same.

Angell had a massive caseload, with some of the worst cases

anywhere. The clientele, who pounded Angell's shoreline like the tide, covered the range of New England's population—from gang members and the homeless of Boston's inner city, to corporate executives, professional sports figures, and popular entertainers. It was a place where interns, some still as fresh of face as teenagers, found maturity quickly or languished.

The hospital provided a professional feast for young doctors who emerged from veterinary school craving to know more. The hungriest interns, those who wanted to see and experience everything and who reluctantly retreated to their shabby dwellings only to sleep, found their skills growing exponentially. The most obsessed believed they had reached nirvana, even years afterward mourning the ending of the internship.

"That internship was a tremendous learning experience," recalled former intern Bud Keller, now a veterinary surgeon in South Carolina. "And it's not so much the medicine or surgery: mainly, it's knowing what you can and can't do. A lot of it is figuring out who you are and what you're capable of.

"People who go through that internship leave there with a tremendous amount of self-confidence, maybe more so than at any other internship, because you're not spoon-fed anything. You're not led around by the hand. You're not part of a service. It's you. And a lot of times it's you against all of Boston."

For her part, Lynne Morris found comfort in the internship, though at times she longed for relaxation, sunny climes, and her fiancé Eric. She had gotten through the early stages with no major problems and in fact was relieved to see how well she had kept her emotions in check.

Then, a few months into the game, she was sitting at home when Eric called from overseas. "I had a really bad week," she remembered. "I put to sleep all these animals. Everything I saw had cancer. I couldn't cure anything. They were all dying. It was terrible. Then I heard Eric's voice on the phone and just started bawling my eyes out. There he is, thousands of miles away; there's nothing he can do. And here I am, crying at five dollars a minute."

ANGELL'S CLIENTELE WAS NOTHING IF NOT A challenge. The interns, who handled most walk-ins, including anything that came in at night, constantly had to adjust to the differences in social strata, intelligence, and temperaments of the area's many pet owners. With new victims perpetually rolling in, seldom did they have time to connect on any personal level.

It didn't help that many clients dismissed the interns because of their youth. "People naturally assume—and probably rightly so—that we don't have a lot of the knowledge and skills of a lot of these vets out there," said intern Gary Block. "But we make up for a lot of that by our commitment and the time we take and the fact that we're nervous as hell about fucking up."

With some interns, a lack of maturity in handling touchy situations was evident. One day when an owner rushed in with his dying dog, an intern snidely remarked that if he had come sooner for its chronic heart disease, perhaps the animal could have been saved. What the young doctor never took a moment to learn was that the man and his wife were devoted owners who had been bringing their pet to an outside veterinarian.

Another time, an intern had grown exasperated and was all but pestering an owner to put his cancer-ridden pet out of its pain. "I lost my father today!" the client finally snapped. "I just can't bring myself to lose my dog, too!"

Yet, the interns had a youthful exuberance and idealism that made them Angell's lifeblood. There were those—Lynne Morris among them—who drove out to a client's home on a day off if the owner had a problem coming in. One female intern from years past was renowned for sitting with grieving owners, holding their hands, and copiously weeping along with them.

And if a dependable client needed a break on a bill, almost every intern knew who the soft touches were in the financial office. Still, Paul Gambardella and his managers waged a never-ending offensive against those who intentionally undercharged owners who were short on cash. While interns were not the only guilty parties, at least every class had one or two who were notorious for working the angles. One previous intern was dubbed "Dr. Giveaway."

It worked like this: a radiograph would be shot, studied, then thrown away, never to appear on the bill. A major procedure would be scribbled in as some less expensive service. Sometimes an intern would cut a needy client a break by intentionally underestimating the cost of treatment, thereby reducing the customer's required down payment. And the number of clients to benefit from shadowy mid-night surgeries will never be known.

Every year at least one intern conducted a covert war to save even pets that management deemed beyond saving. Every now and then, for instance, an owner would bring in a sick dog, ravaged with a deadly parvoviral infection perhaps, and never return, let alone pay the bill. With innumerable healthy pets awaiting adoption in the var-ious shelters, the fate of such an abandoned animal was often euthanasia. A soft-hearted intern might then adopt the dog and, fly-ing in the face of policy, scurry around to find a friend or someone else to take it.

Such behavior could be good for the givers. Angell does offer assistance to its poorest clients—and often makes exceptions for oth-ers—but a number of interns believed it was too little for such a suc-cessful nonprofit. They had accepted the internships hoping to save animal lives and were distressed to find that Angell was run like a business and that many clients who could not pay ended up having their pets euthanized. Helping someone now and then—especially if it involved a touch of skullduggery—was a salve for all the angst, long hours, low pay, and bottom-of-the-barrel work that fell to them.

It was a rationalization that not everyone embraced. "If you're the veterinarian and this is breaking your heart so goddamned bad, come up with some cash," said staff neurologist Allen Sisson. "It's easy to be moralistic with someone else's money. To me, to do what those interns are doing is white-collar crime."

On the other hand, clients didn't always endear themselves to the interns. Some clients had the false impression that the interns were not licensed veterinarians. Others wanted only male doctors to see their pets. There was no predicting how particular visitors regarded their animals and what degree of care they would demand or even be able to afford. On Lynne's first overnight, a man came in with a cocker spaniel that had been hit by a car. The dog was in shock and was suffering from a broken femur and a pneumothorax (air in the chest cavity, probably from a damaged lung). The dog needed to be entered into intensive care immediately and would have to remain for at least a few days. Morris estimated that the bill would run from five hundred to a thousand dollars. *"What?"* burst the owner. "I can go out and buy another dog for five hundred dollars. Why should I fix this one?" The dog was euthanized.

Sometimes the cases in which the animals lived were the most exasperating. One night an insolent young man wearing sunglasses came in with a cat, an old, unexplained burn mark down its side, its bladder the size of a softball. The cat was unable to urinate, and its creatinine level was precariously higher than normal. "It was a urethral obstruction," Morris said, "but it was bad. It had been going on for a long time. He was definitely a candidate for death." On top of that, the guy had no money.

Morris tried to explain about the animal's rapidly declining condition, the limitations of what she could do if the man could not pay, the option of euthanasia. The entire time she was speaking, the fellow kept on his headphones and sunglasses. Now and then, to show he was alive, he nodded. Lynne felt like she was talking to the walls.

When she was finished, the client spoke: "Man, if I was hooked up on life support, I wouldn't want anybody to pull the plug on me. And I *don't* want anybody to pull the plug on my cat."

Fatigued, Morris held her fire. She later told me that at that same moment, a serene image passed through her mind. "I would pull the plug on you," she thought.

5
Brum

LIKE WORKPLACES ACROSS THE COUNTRY, ANGELL
Memorial had its share of Gary Larson's "Far Side" cartoons on display. On the bulletin board behind the receptionist's desk, for
instance, one depicted a dog boasting to another that he was going to
the veterinarian to get *tutored*. In surgery was one that portrayed a
team of Larsonesque doctors huddled around the operating table as
one of the patient's body parts sproinged into the air.

On an office door in a distant corner of the first floor, one
showed an Acme salesman arriving at a would-be customer's house.
Lurking behind a tree in the yard was a typically peculiar-looking
individual. Posted on the fence was a warning: "Beware of Doug."
This particular room, a short walk from the library, was occupied by
ICU's Alicia Faggella and one Douglas Evan Brum. (Because of space
limitations, most of the veterinary staff shared offices.)

Brum's decorative contributions recalled the style of a college
freshman. The top of his desk was always a wreck, covered with
memos, case files, and at least one bizarre toy, be it a doll that dropped
its pants or a toy pig that launched a plastic rotten apple from its

mouth. A bumper sticker on his desk proclaimed, "I'm the person your mother warned you about." Behind his chair the shelves were loaded with empty Jack Daniels bottles. A multicolored hammock, slung on a metal frame and looking like it belonged on a cruise ship, was against one wall. Amidst the veterinary manuals on a ceiling-high bookcase was the twenty-fifth-anniversary *Sports Illustrated* swimsuit issue.

Brum himself had woolly black hair, with a full beard and mustache. If you looked close enough, you could see the scars on his nose and lower lip, permanent reminders of the rottweiler that tore his face one day during an examination.

It was mid-afternoon. For the last hour, Brum had been motoring through Angell's halls, checking on patients and answering a smattering of short questions from interns and anyone else wily enough to catch him on the run. Now, as he sat sorting through a stack of telephone messages, a dozen folders, and intern requests for letters of reference, the telephone rang. On the other end was Nancy Cuddyer, the waiting room coordinator, clearly stressed.

Last week the computers had crashed, leaving staffers to schedule patient visits by pen and paper, without any knowledge of what appointments had already been made. This week the hospital was paying the price. The system was up again, but now many of the twenty-minute appointment slots had been double-, triple-, even quadruple-booked. Some doctors were deluged; others had no appointments for hours.

Some staff doctors flatly refused Cuddyer's pleas to help and take a walk-in or two. Others needed to be cajoled. But Brum, no matter how hellish the waiting room got and no matter how busy he was, never said no. Not just with the overflow cases, either: he also volunteered to see some of the most belligerent owners, figuring he was sparing everyone else the pain. "I hate this woman," he murmured to himself one day as he legged through radiology to see one particularly nasty client. A surgeon looked up, startled. "If *you* hate her, then, man, I don't *ever* want to see her."

To make room for the surprise cases, Brum would juggle his own schedule and, if worse came to worst, work later that night. Five or six small favors a day, combined with his regular work, however, sometimes left him prowling Angell's halls until midnight. His wife and friends grew accustomed to waiting at dinner or various gatherings, sometimes hours after Doug said he would be there.

Now and then, Brum camped at Angell rather than drive home to distant Walpole late at night. On several early morning trips home, he had been so exhausted that he pulled over to the side of the road to sleep. It got to the point that Cuddyer avoided asking him for help; she felt guilty, as if she were taking advantage.

Except, of course, in a pinch. Cuddyer, with no one else willing or able today to see extra patients, desperately wanted someone to treat this one cat. The animal and his owner had come in yesterday, Nancy explained to Brum, simply to have some stitches checked and a drain tube removed from an abscess. The hospital had been bedlam, however, and after more than an hour of forbearance, the woman had to leave. Today she was back and enduring the tedium again.

Brum loped up front, the navy blue neck of his stethoscope draped atop his shoulders. The waiting room was crammed with man and beast; every exam room was in use. Cuddyer pointed out the woman and Doug went over. Introducing himself, he squatted to look briefly at the cat. "I'll be right back," he said, then ran off.

Brum returned with a handful of paper towels, which he spread on the floor as if for a picnic. Then he eased the cat, nervously looking for an escape route, onto his side. "Sometimes I feel like I work at a M.A.S.H. unit," Doug said with a smile, glancing around the crowded room.

The woman laughed out loud. "Incoming!" she sang. "Incoming!"

Brum stroked the animal's coat, quickly examining him. Then he snipped a stitch and slid the tube out. Lickety-split, mission accomplished. He chatted with the woman a minute, advising her when to come back, then scurried off again.

"I'm supposed to have a get-together with some friends," he said, plunging through the waiting room door toward surgery. "More likely it's going to be a midnight get-together."

SUCH WAS LIFE FOR DOUG BRUM. HE WAS LATE FOR, or totally missed, everything from the regular sushi dinners he had with old friends to his Seder at Passover. It wasn't that his caseload was unbearable. Nor did he shun laughter and good times. In truth, he had more close friends and outside interests—from astronomy to hiking—than most people. It was simply that Brum's life tended to be like one giant, all-inclusive painting; sometimes it was hard to see where his work life stopped and personal life began.

To Doug, the hospital was a step or two beyond vet school. He could practice a high level of care, and he had plenty of dedicated friends and cohorts wandering the halls with him. Every day it was something new and fascinating and fun. Brum went from case to case, day to day, with the emotional intensity of someone who had won a free blitz through the supermarket—and they were paying him about $52,000 for the honor. (Recently, one local practice unsuccessfully tried to lure Brum away with a salary that would have been $25,000 more, for much less work.)

His immersion in the hospital was not necessarily good for his personal life and in the long run endangered his life span at the hospital. Doug's wife's being employed at Angell did not necessarily make it easier, although many times they traveled together to and from work. Sue—auburn-haired, athletic, and the more serious-minded of the two—was a laboratory specialist in pathology. Usually, she finished work first and waited, napping on the hammock in Doug's office, reading, or playing with an electronic toy as an intern or client asked him "just one more" question or favor.

It was winter, but Doug and Sue were already looking ahead to September. They had recently gone to their respective supervisors to request that entire month off for vacation. They were planning to travel out West to visit friends and backpack through a variety of national parks. Already they were asking friends who had made similar trips for places to visit. If nothing else, it would be something of a last hurrah for the free-to-go, carefree life of being a young couple without children.

On the surface, no one could detect any great changes in Brum. At work he was as busy as ever. He was director of the intern program. He had recently accepted another quasi-administrative position, which involved setting up the new Wellness Program, Angell's answer to the preventive medicine and client education plans found at human hospitals.

Ever present, though, was the issue of what Doug would do when he and Sue finally started a family. Some staff doctors worked with great efficiency, compartmentalizing their lives to the point that they always went home at a reasonable hour. Others had been swallowed whole by the great whale of Angell, some of them putting in marathon efforts that stretched not over a few weeks or months but years; some of them eventually came home to discover that their children, whom they hardly knew, were packing for college.

Being an Angell veteran, Sue knew all the stories, and of course, she knew her husband. She questioned whether Doug could leave Angell behind and be there for their family. Doug knew she was right, and he would frequently talk to his superiors about finding a balance. He came straight out and told Mike Bernstein, head of medicine: I don't *want* to be like you; I want to have a life outside of this place.

Brum grew up in the affluent New York suburb of Great Neck, on Long Island. His father, Leonard Brum, had made a fortune as a manufacturer of ladies' undergarments—Flora-Lee was the company's name—in Long Island City. He never pushed Doug to get into the family business, but his work ethic rubbed off on the boy.

Doug was raised with few material wishes unfulfilled. He had a spacious backyard, where he and all the neighborhood kids often gathered to play. The Brums traveled a lot. Doug spent a number of summers at an arts camp in Connecticut, first as one of the young charges and later as a counselor. All that he could have asked for growing up was perhaps a few siblings with whom to crash around the nice ranch-style house.

Doug was nine or ten when he started talking about being a veterinarian, a self-fulfilling prophecy. His parents encouraged him, as did some of his relatives. And whenever anyone had an animal question, it was always, "Ask Doug—he's going to be a vet."

A dog and some cats were standards around the Brum house. No rodents ever made it into the house, and Mrs. Brum forbade snakes, but Doug had everything else, from iguanas to tropical fish.

Growing up, Brum's bedroom was a shrine to the animal kingdom. Figurines of everything from lions to serpents were all over. Colorful encyclopedias and other books about animals jammed his bookshelves. His walls were plastered not with posters of rock and roll stars, like those of his friends, but wild animals.

The only exceptions were the magazine cutouts of various players from his favorite professional football team, the Miami Dolphins. One day in ninth grade, Doug's friend Ken Gold asked him why he rooted for the team from Florida, when all their buddies at Great Neck South High School were devoted to the nearby New York Giants or Jets. "Dolphins are the most intelligent sea mammals," Brum replied.

By then Doug was definitely on a veterinary school track. His grades in the sciences were stellar. He spent two summers volunteering at the Animal Medical Center in Manhattan, helping prep animals for surgery and monitoring them in their cages. He received a perfect score on the standardized Advanced Placement Test for college biology.

Gold, now a physician with Harvard's health plan and still one of Brum's closest friends, believed that being an only child was the main reason Doug became so fond of animals, which served as substitutes for siblings. It was also one of the reasons, Gold said, that Brum would become so socially adept; he liked having plenty of happy faces around. Gold, in fact, always suspected that Doug envied him for having three brothers. "Doug used to hang out at my house in high school," Gold said, "and he was adopted to a certain extent because he always wanted some family."

Brum and Gold both went to Union College in Schenectady, New York. At an orientation meeting for freshmen who planned to go on to professional programs in the health sciences, Brum listened to an administrator tick off the grade point averages they would probably need to be accepted into medical and dental school. "And if you want to go to veterinary school," the official said, throwing up his hands, "I don't know what you need. I can't get anybody in!"

That remark was challenge enough to help propel Brum into Cornell's veterinary school. As hard as he labored those eight years of college and vet school, though, Brum always had a playful side, whether he was wearing a cowboy hat and passing out the shot glasses at parties or good-naturedly bedeviling his friends.

After graduation Brum ended up in Angell's internship program, largely because his cousin, today a veterinarian in upstate New York, had been through the program and encouraged Doug to follow suit. On the Saturday of his first long weekend at the hospital, Brum put down six or seven animals, every one as heartrending as the one before it. That was only the beginning. By the end of his internship, he was emotionally and physically spent.

Something about Angell, though, ensnared Brum. He worked at a private practice in northern Massachusetts briefly, grew restless, and quit. He was basically adrift, lounging around the apartment he shared with Sue, whom he met during his internship, when Angell called. There was an opening for a junior staff doctor, a notorious crash-and-burn slot that involved seeing patients by appointments as well as emergencies. It involved weekends, late afternoons, and nights. Brum was wary at first, but once he started, he felt like he was home again.

Now he had been on staff for four years. The place was ideal for his personality. The medicine was challenging; that was important. He also found the hospital liberating, just a step beyond the freedom he knew as a student. He was back to working crazy, draining hours, yet he loved it.

As long as he performed, Brum could be himself. He was a junior staffer with no intentions of becoming a specialist, an attitude that usually would mean a dead end at a specialty hospital like Angell. With Doug, though, it hardly mattered. "They keep me because I have what I think is the Angell spirit," he said. "I know what the place is. I generally don't bitch too much. I work hard. I like what I'm doing. Moralewise, I'm good for the place."

If Angell had an award for bonhomie, Brum would win hands down. As it was, you never quite knew what to expect when you rang back to his desk. Usually, he answered the phone with a simple "Satan's office" or an oily "Hah-lo." With clients and people he did not know well, Brum kept his decorum, but if it was a friend, he could burst forth with "You loser!"

Hospital rules may have forbidden alcohol on the premises, but it would have been hard not to have heard about Brum's famous after-work shots of bourbon with the interns in his office. And when tensions reached their peak, Brum was known to parade into surgery, say, and, to a burst of laughter, simply drop his pants and stand there in his underwear. (To the regret of some people, Brum's antics were fewer in recent years. Management attributed it to a growing maturity; certain co-conspirators thought he had sold out; Brum himself said he was just too damn busy.)

Shenanigans aside, many staffers assumed quite seriously that Brum was being groomed to someday be chief of staff, noting his chumminess with Gambardella and the other powers that be. His officemate, in fact, dubbed him "the Favorite Son."

For his part, Brum had his doubts that he ever would be in line for the job. Moreover, he didn't want it. "I'm trained as a vet, and I want to stay a vet," he said. "I don't want to deal with the big questions and the managerial bullshit. I don't want to lose sight of what I'm good at."

Some predicted that for his own sanity Brum would eventually depart Angell for a quieter practice, where duty wasn't always calling. Even pathologist Jim Carpenter, who saw plenty of places where staffers could work harder, approached Paul Gambardella with his fears. "We have to keep an eye on Doug Brum," he told his boss gravely. "He can do too much; he can harm himself."

Brum may have lacked specialist credentials, but he managed to carve out an unassailable niche. He was always among the top annual income producers, bringing in as much as $450,000 for the hospital in a single year.

Brum had admirable patience, which, was most evident in the types of cases he carried. Doug saw most of the animals with Cushing's disease, an adrenal malfunction requiring weeks, even months, of touch-and-go outpatient therapy that called for both patience and attentiveness from doctor and owner. He had scores of geriatric dogs and cats with everything from renal disease to diabetes. And though Angell had a staff oncologist, Brum treated plenty of patients with cancer.

His specialty was personality, which led one colleague to teasingly dub him "the sensitive, Jewish male doctor." For starters, he was good with pets. "Some animals dislike people," said Sue Brum, "but not many animals dislike Doug." When pets came in, Doug always spent a minute or two petting and playing with them; he spoke to the dog or cat in a peculiar Elmer Fudd voice. (At home the Brums had a twenty-five pound monster cat named Max, who ruled the roost, and a sweet, mixed-breed dog named Sebastian, who regularly fetched the newspaper and smiled on command.)

Carter Luke, the MSPCA's vice president for humane services, was one of a few dozen employees who entrusted their pets to Brum. "He's warm," Luke said of Doug. "He's funny; he's got a smile on his face. He's a constructive, positive person. Do you have any idea how good he is? I don't. God, for all I know, he's a butcher. But people love him."

Some owners wrote him stories and poems about their pets. Often they came bearing gifts, from fruit baskets to fine liquor; one gentleman even presented him with a silver Rolex watch.

Others used their visits to vent their personal woes. One owner, whose dog had a urinary tract infection and various other ailments, wept for half of the appointment. Through sobs she told Brum of her disintegrating marriage and dismal home life. "Thank you, Doctor," she said as she departed. "I know the dog's in better shape than me."

Once when Doug returned from vacation, he was greeted by a fellow veterinarian who reported that in his absence she had tried to assist one of his regulars and her pet. "She told me that Doug Brum is the only veterinarian in the United States," the colleague said, "and that I'm a piece of shit."

Brum's role as director of Angell's internship program gave him authority over more than a dozen young veterinarians. Even then, he was more of a big brother than a boss. To Paul Gambardella's bewilderment, Brum took on the role of number one morale booster, teacher, and shoulder to cry on. "Doug Brum needs to be loved by everybody here," the chief of staff said. "but he's putting too much time into it and he knows it."

Only a few years out of veterinary school himself, Doug was one of the few staff doctors to go out for drinks and dinner with the young veterinarians. Periodically, he would have all of them over to Chez Brum for much-welcomed free food, to splash in the swimming pool, and to play Ping-Pong or Foosball in his basement. At almost every party, Doug would gather them around to watch his favorite horror movie, *The Evil Dead, Part II.*

Brum wanted to show the interns that the program could be more than perpetual angst. A few years ago—after Brum, a handful of interns, and a couple of staff workers had drained Doug's last bottle of bourbon—he convinced a night supervisor that he needed something in MSPCA president Gus Thornton's office. That evening Brum and his merry band made off with a bottle of Dewar's White Label Scotch that Thornton kept for visiting VIPs. "Thank you, Gus," read the note Doug left.

It only followed that the interns one year presented Brum with the annual award for the staff doctor who had helped them the most. When boyhood friend Ken Gold learned of it, he congratulated his pal. "Now do me a favor," he said, pondering all of the extra hours Doug must have put in to make him so beloved. "Promise me you'll never win it again."

6

Anthony

AROUND THE HOSPITAL SOME OF THE LIAISONS AND nurses dubbed Anthony Bonacorso the "Italian Stallion." He and his friends were heavy into sports, from hockey to weight lifting. Dark haired and olive skinned, with thick, powerful arms, twenty-six-year-old Bonacorso cut an imposing figure. Anthony had in fact come home with trophies from a number of amateur bodybuilding competitions. Whenever he walked into Angell, he carried himself with obvious self-confidence.

Yet Bonacorso was in a spin of confusion and worry over his dog Matteo. What's more, his personality was such that he could not sit idly by. Instead, he learned how kidneys work and about the ravaging effects of ethylene glycol. He picked up the phone and cold-called a kidney specialist at powerhouse Massachusetts General Hospital and to ask his opinion. He inquired how a human would be treated under similar circumstances. When he was told about kidney dialysis machines, he asked about buying one. After he learned that he could probably acquire a used one for $20,000, Bonacorso debated making the purchase.

"Fortunately," he later said, "I was in a position where I could absorb a hit like that financially. Actually, I was more prepared to absorb it financially than mentally, because I didn't want to part with my dog."

Initially, Bonacorso struck me as a hard case. He grew up in working-class Winthrop, a tough, little oceanside town near Logan International Airport, and had a rough edge in his speech and manner. At times he seemed to talk *at* you rather than *to* you. Strong minded, he eventually got into a terse exchange with one of the volunteers and a nurse over a delay in visiting Matteo.

Over time, he grew more likable. He showed up one day with a snapshot of Matteo as a puppy wearing a red bandanna. He brought in the dog's favorite toy, an orange ball with a thousand rubbery studs. Even the most hardened Angell staffers had to smile the day that a crowd of Anthony's family and friends, including his aged father, somberly showed up to visit, one by one patting and hugging the dog.

The youngest of three children, Bonacorso had been working with his father, a bridge contractor, since he was fourteen. He paid his own way through three years of classes at Northeastern University in Boston and was now completing his undergraduate degree in finance and marketing at Boston College. He ran his own construction company. Eventually, he would take a stab at starting a small record label, Cathedral Records.

While he was something other than Saint Francis of Assisi, Anthony had a soft heart for creatures. "I don't fear animals," he told me. "My girlfriend will tell you: in many cases animals have come up to me. I've had birds fly right next to me. I've fed squirrels; I fed a raccoon; I fed a skunk. Because I understand that if you put yourself in a neutral position, a nonthreatening position, you will find that animals will respond.

"I had a bird, a white dove, that for some reason flew into my backyard. It was injured or something. I fed it; I took care of it. I used to leave the back door open in my house, and as God is my witness, the bird would come in, eat, fly out during the day, sit up on the roof, and later in the afternoon fly back into the house. The bird did this for about a month. I tell you, this stuff happens to me."

As a boy, he had a sweet Labrador retriever cross, Doobie, who was hit by a car when Anthony was about sixteen. The doctors at Angell pieced the dog together but said he would never again have feeling in his hindquarters. When the family brought the dog home, Anthony ministered to him, bathing him twice daily and even sleeping with him. But in the end, Doobie was too badly hurt; Anthony's parents had him euthanized.

A few years later, when he was nineteen, Bonacorso got Jake. One of his buddies had just gotten the rottweiler puppy but found he had no time for a dog. He only had to ask Anthony once whether he was interested. A rottweiler was just what he wanted. "I'm a very physical person," Bonacorso explained, "very active in sports, aggressive in certain things, but not violent. I just like to do aggressive things. I could never hunt, but I do like to explore nature. I wanted a good outdoors dog that I could have fun with, wrestle with, play ball, Frisbee, whatever."

A rotty seemed ideal. "Call it a macho dog, if you will," he said. "At that time, I probably had a little more of a desire to have a masculine dog. But after I realized what the breed was really about, I fell in love with the breed. They're one of the most intelligent dogs."

Stout, with a massive head, Jake was beautiful. Anthony spent a lot of time with him, and over six years the pair grew close. "I raised that dog in the home with just love," he said. "I exposed it to people at a young age so he wouldn't be fearful of people. I never hit the dog."

Bonacorso even traded in his Corvette for a Jeep Cherokee, the better to ferry around a 140 pound canine. He read up on rotties, their history, and their needs. He learned about proper training and spent lots of time on the ballfields across from his home teaching Jake a variety of commands, none of them having to do with the word attack.

A few years ago, Jake died as a result of gastric torsion, technically known as gastric dilation-volvulus (GDV). No one could say exactly what triggered the dog's stomach to twist on itself. Anthony noted that the dog had done a lot of swimming the day before he died, joining him and his friends on a water-skiing outing. For what it was worth, he also remembered that someone had fed the dog a bagel.

After finding Jake dead in the backyard that morning, Bonacorso brought him to Angell for an autopsy. Pathologist James Carpenter signed off on the case, saying Jake was indeed a victim of GDV, a not-uncommon ailment in large, deep-chested dogs. (Though nothing is definitive, GDV is suspected of being connected to a combination of heavy exercise, excessive water intake, and dry dog food.)

Anthony wrapped his dead dog in a blanket and, inexplicably, an American flag, then buried him six feet underground near the lake on his brother's property, a place the animal seemed to have loved. He put a headstone on the grave as well: "JAKE, MY BEST FRIEND."

Anthony could last only four months without a dog. Then he visited a rottweiler breeder and paid eight hundred dollars for the pick of his latest litter. Unlike the other pups, Matteo was calm, almost timid, suggesting to Anthony an even disposition.

"I remember taking him home the first night," Bonacorso said. "I had a big dog cage, one of those transport cages that you bring on a plane. I had a nice big one for him, and I put him in there. He just cried and cried and would not sleep, so that first night I took him into bed, and he slept with me."

Before he knew it, Anthony was in love again. As with Jake, he brought Matteo to the athletic field near his house and three times a day worked on training. Of the two dogs, Matteo was better disciplined, perhaps because Anthony had grown as a trainer. "I would snap my fingers, and the dog would raise to attention," he recalled. "I taught him 'stay,' 'down,' 'sit,' 'circle,' and 'heel.' He knew both voice and hand commands.

"How many dogs do you know that you could take a piece of steak, put it in his mouth, tell him to stay, and he would not chew it? Not only that, but go one step further and remove it from his mouth. A dog would never do that for anyone unless they had total trust and respect for that master."

Like Jake, Matteo too became Anthony's sidekick. Once, he rented an RV and drove out to California with the dog, exploring the coast together for a few weeks before his girlfriend joined them. He told of descending and climbing a one-hundred-and-fifty-foot cliff with the dog, a harrowing proposition if the animal—or human—was the least bit skittish. "At times I would have to physically pick him up and press him over my head and put him on the next section," said Anthony. "He had that much trust in me."

Now, as his dog lay glumly in intensive care, Anthony thought back over all the good times. He spoke of loyalty and respect and how those concepts manifested themselves perfectly in a dog. "A dog is so unselfish," he told me when things looked worst. "He'll stay with his master until the end. If I was in danger, Matteo would stay with me."

It was obvious what Bonacorso was thinking: He and Matteo were on a two-way street. He simply could not give up hope.

7
Carp

JIM CARPENTER WAS A WEED. AT LEAST THAT IS HOW the head of pathology had come to see himself at Angell Memorial Animal Hospital. "Do you know the definition of a weed?" he liked to ask. "A weed is a plant out of place." Even the loveliest flower, he explained, might be considered a weed were it to sprout at the wrong time or in the wrong location, such as on a putting green or through a crack in a city sidewalk.

Taking appearances alone, Carpenter would have fit in best on a smoky battlefield of the Civil War. He looked the part of a general of that era, with his unruly salt-and-pepper mustache and beard, graying hair, and a squarish head just larger than average.

He had the ability to lock his mind onto whatever work was at hand, with the result being a visage that was often a study in fierce determination. The look was disconcerting to some, particularly the youngest members of the staff, who worried about who might or might not like them. It did not help that Carpenter stood a hefty six-foot-two and weighed 230 pounds.

Yet something about Carpenter's features failed to fit the intim-

51

idating bill: often hidden by the eyepieces of his microscope and his sporadically worn glasses were the clearest light blue eyes. They were giveaways to a genial side of his nature.

His fifty-seventh birthday was in March. As Carpenter entered his thirty-second year at Angell, he was the senior doctor on staff as well as the longest running hospital employee. He also commanded the largest salary—close to $114,000 at its peak. At the time, he pulled in more than Gambardella and esteemed cardiologist Neil Harpster. In fact, Jim's longevity and skills had made him the third highest compensated person in the entire MSPCA.

Carpenter had begun as an intern, stayed on as a clinician for a decade, then shifted gears and became a pathologist. In the entire organization, only Thornton and one or two others went back further.

His home away from home was the basement of Angell, which was divided between pathology, the hospital laundry, and purchasing. Space was at a premium; when it finally ran out in his section, Carpenter began housing old slides and specimens in army green filing cabinets in the hall. When the ancient pipes overhead began to leak like the biblical Flood, Carpenter's people simply gathered their papers and slides from their offices, set up camp on dry ground, and returned to their labors.

Not much daunted Jim Carpenter or, as a result, his workers. Weeds of course sprout under all kinds of conditions.

Carpenter was a department head, so he spent much of his time managing. He oversaw a department that employed as many as fifteen people, including supervisors, technicians, and support staff, in both clinical pathology and histopathology. His greatest value to Angell, however, was his own ability to diagnose hundreds of tissue samples sent from the veterinarians upstairs and elsewhere.

As the new year began, he was also hard at completing a paper with a colleague from the Midwest. "It's going to be the best manuscript on feline toxoplasmosis in the world," Carpenter said, beaming, "and I will be able to say to myself with some satisfaction that I've seen more lesions of toxoplasmosis in cats than anyone else."

Singular though it may have seemed to outsiders, such was the stuff that brought a merry expression to Carpenter's face and helped establish his eminence as an anatomical pathologist. Many of his veterinary peers, in fact, considered him without equal. Combined with Angell's steady supply of interesting samples, Carpenter's zealous work ethic made it inevitable. Ten years as a practicing veterinarian—the life span of many pets—had only refined his diagnostic abilities, teaching him the real-life possibilities and probabilities of disease.

Carpenter's name was regularly seen in the professional journals, contributing to the field and feeding his hunger for recognition. He discovered numerous small-animal diseases. He was regarded as a dynamic lecturer and teacher. He received tissue samples from all over the country, be it the National Zoo or a veterinarian on the West Coast seeking his expertise.

Still, Carpenter felt like a "plant out of place." The reasons had less to do with his workload than with the changes the years had brought to Angell and the profession. When he arrived in the early 1960s, Angell Memorial Animal Hospital's star was near its zenith. By the 1930s and 1940s, while much of the field was still focused on large animals, Angell's doctors had become expert in treating dogs and cats. Often the veterinarians traded information with some of Boston's best M.D.s, many of whom worked in the immediate area at Harvard Medical School and some of the powerhouse hospitals. Thus, Angell ushered in advancements in surgery, radiology, and reporting previously unknown diseases. Angell also had veterinarians and nurses on duty around the clock, not to mention its unique internship.

When Jim Carpenter got there, Angell was a veterinary mecca. A hybrid, it pulled together some of the teaching aspects of veterinary school with the workload of a gigantic private practice. The staff wrote for prestigious journals, authored books, and lectured far and wide.

Reflecting the era, Angell's veterinarians were usually dressed all in white. The male doctors, who dominated the staff, wore ties at all times. If an intern's shoes—required white bucks—were scuffed, he might well be summoned to the chief of staff's office and ordered to polish them posthaste.

With specialization years away, the staff developed a certain kinship as well. Some of that spirit was a necessary result of working in the tight quarters of the old hospital on Boston's Longwood Avenue. Some of it was facilitated by having a common gathering place, a first floor conference room, where the doctors ate lunch together, swapped thoughts on cases, and took in seminars.

It was an environment where young Carpenter thrived. When he came for his internship, he was twenty-five years old, a Wisconsin native who had never been farther from home than Iowa, where he attended veterinary school. It was pouring rain when Carpenter and his wife, Grace, accompanied by their wailing infant daughter, rolled into town in an old Pontiac sedan with broken windshield wipers and three hundred dollars to their names.

Carpenter came into the internship with a reputation as a stellar student. He had ranked first in his class in high school as well as at the University of Wisconsin's College of Agriculture and Iowa State University's veterinary school.

Yet, when he arrived at Angell, he was anything but overly confident. In truth, he was anxious and awestruck just to be there. For his first few days, Carpenter's innards were churning. His first patient was a young springer spaniel with bloody feces, a routine enough matter. After he did the physical exam, however, Carpenter's mind went blank. His adviser, Dr. Midge Petrak, then asked him to join her in the hallway. Carpenter recalled, "We stepped out of the room, and she says, 'You know, parasites are a common problem. Now, what parasite could cause blood in the stool?' Well, shit, I knew hookworms, but I couldn't even think of it, for God's sake."

His torment carried over to the bane of every Angell intern—overnight duty. Like today's, the nighttime interns of Carpenter's day were sometimes granted a few hours to sleep, if business slowed. At the old building, they bedded down in a cramped room on the second floor. When an emergency arose, the hospital supervisor clicked across the courtyard and up a flight of stairs to rouse the young doctors.

Carpenter usually was already awake. "I could always hear the supervisor's footsteps coming," he said. "He didn't have to make the stairs, that's how hyper I was. I was so concerned about whether I'd be able to take care of the problem. That's what I remember the most: the unknown problem. The unknown was what worried me."

Carpenter had hoped to win a pathology residency at the hospital, but for some reason he was rejected. Instead, chief of staff Gerry Schnelle offered him a job as a staff veterinarian.

His stature as a clinician grew with each year. Many clients became Carpenter loyalists. After all, he was talented. Perhaps more important to the hospital administration, though, was that he came in early, worked during lunch, and left late. Not uncommon for the day, he also doubled as a surgeon and assisted in interpreting many of the X rays for the staff. Carpenter spent countless hours following up on his patients that died, performing autopsy after autopsy to see first-hand whether his opinions had been correct.

He also developed uncanny skills of palpation, examination by touch. It was a highly respected art, but one that lost some luster with the onset of better imaging technology and laboratory tests. "Probably the person with the best palpation skills that I ever knew here was Jim Carpenter," said staff dermatologist Richard Anderson, a former intern. "He could literally feel an ovary on a dog, which I don't think anybody here today can do."

"When I came here, he was *the* clinician," added cardiologist Harpster. "He was the man that had all the answers."

Carpenter attributed his skills to plain hard work. Others believed he was blessed with an innate ability to take an animal's condition and medical history, pull them together with his own experience and intuition, and come up with a sound diagnosis even when others were stumped. "He could go along a course, a thought pattern, and be innovative and come up with the difficult answer, the not-obvious answer," said Gus Thornton. "That is what sets apart the truly great clinician."

Carp, as he was known, brought to Angell an individualism and a work ethic that recalled another age. He was also so principled that he resisted when higher-ups suggested he pay famous or wealthy clients certain attentions not given the average customer. Sometimes when his medical opinion clashed with a client's wishes, he would argue vociferously. Some of that was immaturity. What was obvious was that he cared—passionately.

Carpenter was also long-suffering, no small quality at an animal hospital with Angell's diverse clientele. One Christmas Eve in the sixties, he was working the late shift, when in staggered a fellow in his mid-fifties, dressed in threadbare clothes, with a ragged beard and a mustache. At his side was a black-and-white mongrel with anal sac disease. It was a common problem, especially in small dogs, and Carpenter went about his job of manually expressing the vestigial glands, which can fill with a bitter-smelling fluid.

"I bet you think I can't pay for this appointment!" the man roared. He had obviously been drinking.

Carpenter looked up. "No," he said, "that's not my responsibility. I just take care of the medical aspects of the visit. I have nothing to do with the finances."

"Well, I *still* bet you think I can't pay for it." The man fished from his pocket the greatest wad of cash Carpenter ever saw—hundred-dollar bills galore. The veterinarian stared in disbelief as the man flipped through the cash, once and forever establishing his solvency.

Then he suddenly demanded that Carpenter listen up. He had a song in his head, and he insisted that the doctor hear it—in its entirety. With that, he began warbling "The Yellow Rose of Texas."

"It was the most uncomfortable thing for me to be in this room with that dog and that client and to have him sing the *whole* song," Carpenter would later say with a laugh. "I did it, but it was the longest song I ever listened to."

On another occasion an older couple from Rhode Island brought in a twelve-year-old parakeet with nodules all along its claws, some of them oozing a white matter. Unsure of what he was seeing, Carpenter consulted Midge Petrak, the avian specialist. She in turn looked the bird over; outside the exam room, she informed Jim that this was a classic case of gout.

"So I went back into the room," Carpenter recalled, "and I said, 'Dr. Petrak and I feel confident that the bird has gout.' And just as soon as I said that, it was the only time in my life I have ever heard a parakeet talk, that bird said, *'Shit.'*

"After I recovered from the shock, I said, 'Wow, I've never heard a parakeet talk.' And they told me it could say fifteen words; it said 'kiss' and some others. But the one word they were not proud of was 'shit.'"

Carpenter toiled through the sixties. He was so anxious to please his bosses and his clients and to do right by the animals that it became impossible to please everyone. Moreover, he hated to go home with something left incomplete. So he worked. And worked. Finally the beast turned and bit him. Coming to work now became a test of his iron will. "It got to the point that I would just walk into the building, and I could notice the difference in heart rate and respiration," he said years later.

Clients, unable to make short-notice appointments with their favorite veterinarian, became nasty. Often Carpenter was unavailable even for a brief question. Carpenter's professional life was hurtling toward a crisis point. Somehow, things had to change.

That was when he turned to pathology. Over the years, Jim had silently envied the many Angell interns who went on to residencies and careers analyzing tissue and lab work. Now he also wanted in—to learn what pathology had to teach him, but also for safe haven.

Luckily, then Chief of Staff Thornton was open to the idea. Change was under way in the pathology department as it was. He granted Carpenter the time for a residency, then bestowed him with the authority to run the department even before he became board certified.

"My perception was that he needed new mountains to climb," Thornton said. "I think he had done it in clinical medicine and in some ways felt himself at his peak. He has to be constantly challenged, constantly learning. He perceived that wasn't going to happen over the next twenty years if he stayed in clinical medicine.

"Now I also think what he didn't perceive was what was going to happen in those same twenty years to clinical medicine, the sophistication that would have challenged him to keep up. But at the time, he saw pathology as a whole new area that would really challenge him to learn."

The decades passed. Now Jim Carpenter looked around Angell, and nothing was the same. His mentors and closest friends were gone, many of them dead. "I've lost all my heroes," he would say. "I don't have a hero on the staff."

With growing irritability, he saw a hospital where few doctors published with any regularity. He noted with displeasure that staff members straggled in late for meetings. Carpenter was appalled that every doctor's appointment book was not filled weeks in advance. He was frustrated that Angell had no firm position on any number of new issues being debated in veterinary circles, such as whether pets should be vaccinated against Lyme disease. "Times have changed," Carpenter said with a sigh. "My bosses have told me that several times, that I'm not with it."

In many ways, he was the conscience of Angell, the plaintive voice of a day gone by. "Last year I spoke at the American Academy of Veterinary Dermatologists meeting in Scottsdale, Arizona," he said. "And someone walked up to me and said, 'Where is Angell?' What the hell has happened to us? There was a time when *everyone* knew where Angell Memorial Animal Hospital was!"

Carpenter's superiors would tell him that he saw a world of black and white. Too often, they felt, Jim turned a complicated question into a simple matter of moral right or wrong. One veterinarian said that arguing with Jim was like arguing against God or country. "Gray is just a color that is not in his spectrum," Gus Thornton said.

Never shy, Carp would level his cannons at Paul Gambardella, whom he beseeched to be a *leader*, like those of the days of yore. In memos and meetings, he took it as his duty to challenge his boss. Gambardella, for his part, regarded many of the salvos as patronizing, an attempt by someone nearly ten years his senior to diminish him. Carpenter didn't want the chief of staff job, Paul thought; he wanted deference.

"Jim Carpenter has kept me honest," Gambardella said diplomatically. "He's the only department head that can churn my guts. I expect that Jim is going to be up-front and totally honest, and he's going to say what's on his mind, not what he thinks I want to hear. In other words, I don't intimidate Jim, so he feels he can say what he wants. Now, *you* wouldn't call your boss a jerk. Jim would."

In truth, that was not Carpenter's style. More typically, his criticism would be couched within a question, such as "Does *anyone* in this building have the authority or the intestinal fortitude to make decisions for the good of everybody?"

Carpenter had an abiding love for Angell Memorial Animal Hospital. He continued to summon an enthusiasm for his work that could shame people twenty or thirty years his junior. His department was probably the most productive in the hospital. In the end, though, he was discouraged. Retirement, he noted with some relief, was not far away.

"With Dr. Carpenter, you're seeing the last of a dying breed," staff doctor Allen Sisson told me one day. "He's one of the last of what Angell was and will never be again."

8

Decision

ALMOST A WEEK HAD PASSED SINCE MATTEO'S ARRIVAL.
The gray Boston winter deepened. None of Angell's staff was betting
on the dog's survival. He still had not urinated. He sat hunched over
and drooling in a run by the ICU entrance. The skin around his eyes
drooped. He struggled to keep his head raised. A white, plastic
Elizabethan collar, resembling a lampshade, was strapped around his
neck and head to keep him from gnawing at his catheter. He looked
like a sad flower.

When he first came in, Matteo had rumbled at the nurses. Now
he was too lethargic to pay them much heed when they went to feed
him or change his intravenous fluids. "Even a cat would beat you up
now," Anthony told him.

The nurses had grown fond of the dog in the few days he was
there. The doctors were always in and out, but the nursing staff, like
their counterparts in the human field, spent the most time with the
patients. It did not take long for them to pick up on an animal's
behaviors and moods. Now and then they would go in and stroke
Matteo's sleek coat and talk quietly to him.

Around six o'clock on Wednesday night, Bonacorso came to visit. Morris, dreading the moment, stepped into the run and squatted next to him. "I've got bad news," she said. Subdued, she explained what pathologist Carpenter had reported earlier that day. The microscopic tubules of the kidney were essentially plugged with crystals, and the cells around them were sloughing off, making it impossible for the dog to produce urine. In other words, the damage was done. It was, Carpenter had told Morris, the worst case of ethylene glycol poisoning he had seen in his two decades as a pathologist. "If this was my dog," he had said firmly, "I would put it to sleep immediately."

Anthony hugged Matteo. "I can't talk right now," he said.

Morris left Anthony alone. A moment later she rushed over to help a fellow intern with another calamity, a dog newly hit by a car.

Anthony chose to follow Lynne's advice and have his dog euthanized. Matteo's only hope, Anthony knew, as he took Matteo for what he assumed would be their last walk, was if the animal would urinate. "If he pees right now," Bonacorso told a weight lifting friend, who had come for moral support, "it will be a sign from God."

Three seconds later Matteo trickled a bit, took a few steps, raised his leg, and let loose a long stream on a concrete block. "Lynne! Lynne!" shouted Anthony as he hurried down the hall, dog at his side. "He peed! He peed!"

"It was a good beer pee, too!" added his buddy. "Like he had four or five Buds!"

Morris could hardly believe it. She finished what she was doing and went with them to see whether Matteo would perform again. They walked down the hall from intensive care, past the wards, and out into the wintry night. "I'm on a roller coaster right now," Anthony said, talking to the dog. "Two minutes ago you were dead. Now—"

"You *have* to get better," said his friend. "We're not getting good workouts because of you."

They slowly padded around in the cold, beneath the outdoor lights. The dog had a bounce to his step. He seemed resurrected. Again he urinated to beat the band.

"All right," Morris said, "that's pee. I'm convinced; I'm definitely more encouraged." If this continued, she said, there was a chance.

Hope was renewed. Two weeks into the ordeal, Anthony was filled with new enthusiasm. He now seriously debated laying out the $20,000 that a used kidney dialysis machine would cost. He considered possibly flying the dog to a university or someplace else that was experimenting with canine kidney transplants.

Then someone brought up the possibility of using a kidney dialysis machine at Boston's Beth Israel Hospital. At that, disbelief fell across Alicia Faggella's face. It was true that a local imaging facility allowed Angell to rent time for animals on its CAT scanner as well as the nuclear magnetic resonance equipment. The idea of Matteo showing up at a major medical center, however, was getting a little outlandish. "I seriously doubt that they're gonna let a *rottweiler* walk in there with all of those compromised people around," Faggella said.

In the end, it was all talk, anyway: Matteo's performance of that Wednesday night was never repeated. "We think that it was probably one last *umph* from the kidneys," said Morris, "maybe some residual urine that was in the bladder, or the last cells in the kidney were able to squeeze out a few drops of urine."

By the weekend the dog was more depressed than ever. Meanwhile, some nurses and others around the hospital began making remarks that this had gone too far, that Matteo's race had been run. "I don't like to see this," complained one worker in surgery. "The dog's not going to get better, and everyone sees it."

That weekend Bonacorso agreed. Euthanasia had never been far from his mind, but Sunday he took Matteo for a walk, hoping for urine again, and got just a bit. The animal also retched a mouthful of blood. "This is no life for a dog," Bonacorso said.

A gaggle of the young man's friends and family members had come to say good-bye to Matteo. Lynne was off that day. Her friend and fellow intern Beth Campbell would administer the blue barbiturate solution known commercially as Fatal Plus.

Anthony sat on the floor in intensive care, holding Matteo's head in his lap while the dog licked at his face. The dog pulled away when Campbell went to insert the needle. Bonacorso assured him that it was all right, and the job was done.

When it was over, Bonacorso wrapped his arms around Matteo's body. Then, through moist, reddened eyes, he looked around. All of the intensive care nurses were in tears.

Sometimes people on the outside will say, "Gee, you performed a miracle." I've had people come up to me and hug me and say that. I don't think it's a miracle. I think it's a lot of very tired people, who are very poorly paid, doing a lot of hard work—except for my boss, of course, who sits on her fat ass and takes all the credit.

—STAFFER, Angell Memorial Animal Hospital

9

Incoming

EACH DAY AN AVERAGE OF 110 PETS MAKE THEIR WAY
up the long concrete ramp, through two automatic doors, and into
the lobby at 350 South Huntington Avenue. As often as not, the animals come helpless and scared, their owners hoping that within this
building will be an end to pain for their pets.

About 70 percent of the patients are dogs, 28 percent cats, with
the remainder being birds and what are known as "exotics," ferrets,
for example, or lizards.

They come mainly from around Boston and the rest of New
England. It is not unusual, though, for someone to drive from other
venues, Canada, perhaps, or New York. Stories are told of patients fly-
ing out of London on the Concorde and out of Washington, D.C., on
military jets. Staffers speak of Rolls Royces and stretch limousines "as
long as this building" rolling into the parking lot.

Some clients simply arrive on foot. When asked for his address,
one gentleman, injured cat tucked under his arm, replied, "Under the
Fifth Street bridge."

The animals themselves enter in many fashions. Some drag

their owners; others are dragged. Some trundle in on gurneys, others in baby strollers. They come incarcerated in plastic crates known as Pet Taxis or Pet Waggin's. Others disembark from Johnny Walker Red cartons or shoe boxes or gym bags. Often they are cradled, wrapped in baby blankets, beach towels, and, on at least one occasion, a Pierre Cardin shirt. Sometimes a small pet shows up in a paper bag, in a jacket pocket, or with its head peering out from the top of a zippered coat like a brooch.

Some bear names like Fluffy and Kitty and Fido and Rover—commoners, no doubt. But there are also a good number of Princes and Princesses, Dukes and Duchesses, and Kings and Queenies. Perhaps more revealing of their masters' temperaments than of their own, the pets also have names like Sunshine and Smiley as well as Rage and Riot, not to mention Killer and Slaughter.

The most recognizable names, however, usually belong to the owners. In 1975 Elvis Presley had his ten-month-old chow, named Getlo, flown up to Boston on the singer's private Lear jet with a cadre of attendants. At three-thirty one morning, unannounced, an outside veterinarian and a physician ushered the tan-colored female into Angell. The overnight intern ran blood tests and administered medication. Despite the veterinarian's belief that Getlo needed to be admitted, Presley's people elected to the contrary, apparently planning to treat her on their own. She died at Graceland a few months later.

These days most of the celebrities that come in with their pets are from New England. Inevitably, they cause a parade of staffers to happen by the clinic—slowly, time and again.

Doug Brum finally pulled down a blind on the exam room door when curious employees and clients kept peering in at Tracy Chapman and her dachshund, Ginger, who came to be examined before traveling with the popular singer. Another time, Brum had no idea he had seen anyone famous until Joey McIntyre of the then red-hot New Kids on the Block and his beagle, Paris, in for puppy shots, had already departed.

About ten years ago, Paul Gambardella performed delicate disk surgery on a dachshund, Minnie, who belonged to Jimmy Rodgers, then an assistant coach with professional basketball's Boston Celtics. Paul developed a friendship with Rodgers, who went on to head coaching jobs with the Celtics and the Minnesota Timberwolves. Every now and then Rodgers would call him at home with questions about Minnie. Periodically, Gambardella found himself and his wife, Susie, with seats so close to the court in the sold-out Boston Garden that they could see the sweat on their beloved Celtics.

Another time, Gambardella repaired the fractured jaw of Cozette, a silver teacup poodle, the pride and joy of General D'Wayne Gray, then commandant of the United States Marine Corps, and his wife. Paul recalled the incongruity of seeing Gray, the very picture of a hard-bitten Marine, "slobbering" over the tiny poodle and inquiring with heartfelt concern about the animal's condition. Soon afterward Gambardella happened to see a segment on television about the four-star general, including footage of Gray inspecting his men, fear written across their young faces. Gambardella smiled. "I could tell those troops a thing or two about this Marine Corps commandant," he said.

It was the *animals,* however, that many at Angell would have liked to hear talking. Some wondered what secrets were held by Chevron, the Doberman pinscher that belonged to the late New England Mafia boss Raymond Patriarca. The dog was brought to Angell from Rhode Island for a neurologic workup back in 1980. ("Dog is a pet," someone scrawled across his record, "but has had attack training.") What secrets were held by Anka, the rotty belonging to now-imprisoned Raymond, Jr., heir to the Family business? The animal died at the hospital of a ruptured gastric ulcer.

Another visitor was Haylen, a Shih Tzu owned by one Pamela Smart. Before winning tabloid television infamy and a lifelong prison term, Smart devotedly brought the dog down from New Hampshire to be evaluated for allergies. Pamela, a school system employee, so adored Haylen that she instructed her sixteen-year-old lover to put him in her basement—to avoid traumatizing the pooch—while he and a buddy executed her husband.

Stephen King, meanwhile, traveled to Angell from Bangor,

Maine, with his Welsh corgi, Marlowe, who had hip dysplasia. The author was greeted by curious employees and others seeking autographs. One of the denizens of the front desk even proposed that King write a horror story set in an animal hospital like Angell. "You can name it after me," she gushed, *"Esther."*

Waiting room coordinator Nancy Cuddyer, not easily impressed, opted to treat King like any client. "So how are you doing today?" she asked casually when he came over to check in.

"A better question would be 'How is *Marlowe* doing?'" came the reply.

Angell's visitors, whatever their renown, have a wide range of sensibilities about their pets. The majority, of course, have healthy bonds. The dog or cat or whatever is a member of the family, a valued companion, but within the hazy bounds of reason. To many, that includes spending thousands of dollars for treatment if the pet gets sick, or stretching out for the night on a waiting room bench until knowing whether the animal is out of danger.

Veterinarian Alicia Faggella recalled one gentleman who came in with his dog, which had been run over by a car. A leg was broken, and air had escaped from the lungs into the dog's chest. The owner was inconsolable as Faggella tried to explain the injuries in layman's terms. "This may be of some help to you," the man finally said, between sobs. "In real life, I do function as a surgeon."

Others are concerned about their pets' being away from home. Often an owner will ask the veterinarian to take Bowser's special blanket or favorite toy, for example, to put in the cage. One client handed over a tape of positive thoughts, which she asked an intern to play for her recovering feline. Another owner prepared a tape from her entire family talking, so their cat would not be lonely. "Hi, Ginger!" it began. "Mommy's here. Daddy's here, too." Then a whisper: "Say something."

"Hi, Ginger," said an unenthusiastic male voice.

"Be nicer!"

"Hi, Ginger!"

One of Doug Brum's clients, meanwhile, produced a *Caretaker's*

Manual for her cat, which she expected the veterinarian to read. Included were illustrations, a ten-page biography of the cat, its medical history, and its vocabulary ("Loud meow or bloodcurdling meow: 'Please refresh my water.'").

It is true that many owners show up at the hospital only when their animals are all but beyond the pale. For plenty of others, however, it takes only the slightest sign of illness to come sweeping through Angell's doors. A single vomit from little Pepe may have its owner panicked and sitting anxious in the waiting room, day or night.

Once Brum had a woman demand that he draw blood from her dog and test it, though the animal showed no indications of sickness. When she refused to listen to reason, he complied, mostly for her peace of mind. As he predicted, Brum found nothing unusual—with the animal.

As bizarre as some clients seem, their behavior usually has an explanation: sometimes the animal is a person's only connection to a lost loved one or happier days. Sometimes a pet is an unstable individual's sole tie to reality. Sometimes it is a surrogate child for a person or couple who never had offspring. And sometimes fate causes both owner and pet to be combatting the same disease—cancer for example—simultaneously; to give up on the animal would be like giving up on oneself.

Clients would occasionally threaten suicide if their pets were to die, but no one at Angell recalled anyone following through. Doug Brum, though, had spent hours on the telephone with people's psychologists, and he had suggested that a few others seek help. The hospital itself referred clients to a social worker who ran grief-counseling sessions for pet owners.

"I've had people tell me, 'That dog is more important to me than my daughter,'" said Jean Duddy, a staff veterinarian, "and they're not kidding."

One client brought in a dog, dead for days, and asked the doctors to revive it. Another snatched her dead cat and barreled screaming through Angell's halls before holing up in a room for hours. In a ritual only they fully understood, one couple tossed handfuls of glitter around the hospital while their sick pet lay dying in intensive care.

"I feel guilty sometimes," said surgeon Jim Boulay. "People will come in, and they're willing to spend two thousand dollars on their dog in a snap of their fingers. But then they go downtown and walk by a homeless guy and not even give him a second thought.

"Sometimes you want to tell them, 'Look, you need to get a life. This is a dog we're talking about. You're keeping him alive for your own benefit way past when it should be dead.'

"It's a sad commentary on society when people have no friends and come to you and say, 'If I lose this dog, I'll have no warm thing to touch.' That makes you want to cry, that someone can live in the world today and have nobody that gives them any special attention except their dog. That's a sad, sad world."

AS WITH HUMANS, THE RANGE OF MEDICAL WOES FOR animals is tremendous. Many veterinary clinics, Angell included, see scores of vomiting dogs, and cats with urethral obstructions. Also typical are flea-bitten dogs that have gone too far with self-treatment plans, suffering raw "hot spots" on their bodies.

Angell is often the last resort, a place owners come with the toughest, most complicated cases: cancer, heart disease, neurological problems—the list goes on and on. The subjects of pathologist Jim Carpenter's studies alone—from feline panleukopenia to bilateral trigeminal nerve paralysis and Horner's syndrome associated with myelomonocytic neoplasia in a dog—only begin to reveal the depth and complexity of potential ailments.

Laying blame is often impossible. Granted, many illnesses can be traced to breeding; German shepherds, for instance, are prone to certain cancers. But life itself is a risk factor. "We are designed to deteriorate and die," Carpenter said one day, "and you can do it in so many ways. That's the amazing thing, how many things can go wrong."

Then there is trauma. Sometimes animals do unto one another. Cats come in gouged from late-night skirmishes with fellow cats at the garbage cans. A canine battle for dominance might leave one or both participants bowed and bloody.

Sometimes people do unto animals. While the police and human emergency rooms see the daily inhumanity people inflict on one another, Angell—and the MSPCA's law enforcement division—sees creatures that have been poisoned, ensnared in leghold traps, shot, knived, pierced with arrows, starved, and even sexually abused.

Emergency room personnel in human hospitals see firsthand the folly of driving while intoxicated or without a seat belt. At Angell what everyone knows best are the tragedies that stem from letting pets run free. Most obviously, pets are hit by cars, "HBC" in the medical records and "heavy-metal disease" in the black-humor parlance of one veterinarian.

"He never did that before," an owner invariably says as he recounts why Butchie was off his leash when he dashed into the grill-work of a '79 Volaré. One canine car chaser—a tire-biting English bulldog—was drubbed three times, all within six months, and each time was pieced together by an increasingly befuddled Paul Gambardella.

Cats, meanwhile, are brought in with shattered limbs and internal injuries when they survive plunges from rooftops and balconies—chasing birds or insects, no doubt. This is known as "high-rise syndrome."

When Arlyne Koopmann, a secretary in Paul Gambardella's office, one day warned a driver about letting his dog ride in the bed of his pickup, she was curtly rebuffed: "He likes it."

Koopmann was beside herself. "'He *likes* it'?" she echoed later. "There are a lot of things that dog would probably 'like' to do. He'd probably 'like' to go to Las Vegas, if the guy would let him."

Sometimes, though, bad luck just comes knocking. A puppy would be trod upon, or singed after chewing an electrical cord. A cat might doze off in the dryer and wake up sharing a hot spin with the linens. One feline had its head wedged in a drain. A bird was sucked into a vacuum cleaner. Ask any parent: stuff happens.

Nothing, though, seems as common as dogs and cats unable to disgorge objects—"foreign bodies"—that they should have left alone in the first place. As with toddlers, anything and everything is edible if it fits in their mouths.

Some situations sound comic, but foreign bodies often kill. They have the potential to block the digestive tract or perforate the colon beyond repair. Speedy action often makes the difference between life and death.

An abbreviated list of things removed from Angell's patients— through surgery, endoscopy, or induced vomiting—includes combination locks, rocks, panty hose, tampons, garter belts, jewelry, string, golf balls, balls, pacifiers, needles, thread, underpants, ornaments, tinsel, teriyaki sticks, razor blades, steel wool, rubber gloves, emery boards, perfume bottles, as well as hooks, lines, and sinkers.

Hospital staffers also remembered a man and woman who came in and admitted sheepishly that their dog had gobbled their stash of marijuana.

Paul Gambardella once operated on a baby harbor seal— Peniquid, from the New England Aquarium—that had stopped eating. Opening its belly, Paul found 297 coins and a slug—$8.37. Aquarium visitors had tossed them into the animal's pool as if it were a wishing well, and Peniquid simply ate them.

One surgeon told of the time she saw a little metal gorilla, in a pose that looked like it was waving, on the X ray of one patient's belly.

During the holidays Lynne Morris scanned a radiograph of a cat and saw the unmistakable image of a jingle bell. "His mom did a lot of crafts," the intern explained. "If only I had shaken him, I could have made the diagnosis right away."

10 Waiting

THE INTERNS CHRISTENED NANCY CUDDYER "THE
Woman in Black" because she had a penchant for dark clothes. A better nickname might have been "the Air Traffic Controller."

"Hey, roll 'em up!" you could hear her imploring clients on any
given day. A curious German shepherd, tugging on a leash the length
of the waiting room itself, would be panting in front of an elderly
woman, who would be struggling to keep her cat—eyes wide, back
arched—from bolting her arms. "Would you *please* roll up your dog?"

Cuddyer was the waiting room coordinator. She was thirty-
seven years old, with pulled-back, brown-blond hair, a slim build, and
a touch of the streets in her voice.

She had grown up in Jamaica Plain, in a family that overflowed
with boys, and still called the neighborhood home. She walked to
work, in fact, and periodically would recount her adventures on her
journey, near-misses with one menacing character or another. "Yeah,"
she would say matter-of-factly, "they almost got me today."

She was going on her thirteenth year at Angell. In that time she
had seen all kinds of creatures and all kinds of maladies, the worst

being a Doberman pinscher that arrived sliced head to tail by a maniac with a machete.

Another one she never forgot was Sunshine, a beautiful Pekinese crossbreed that three kids held before her one day. "My dog's sick," said one of them, handing him over.

"So I take it to bring it back," Cuddyer recalled, "and it smelled like bug spray. I said, 'Did you spray this dog with something?' The kid says, 'Well, yeah, he had fleas; so we sprayed him.' They had gotten insecticide and sprayed it on that poor dog. But he turned out okay.

"And do you know what? That dog was back here a month later dead. Someone had kicked it to death. Sunshine, poor Sunshine."

Animals had been Cuddyer's love since childhood. She spent countless hours watching television shows like "Lassie" and "The Littlest Hobo." The latter was a series in which a German shepherd, London, rambled around, helping folks in trouble and then padding off into the sunset. As a girl, Nancy never quite accepted the premise. "Oh, no!" she would cry as each episode drew to a close. "He's leaving again!"

One of her first experiences with Angell was at age thirteen, when she came in with her mixed-breed dog, Jack. His jaw was broken, and Nancy had no money. A woman in the front office told her that without funds she should consider euthanasia.

Cuddyer snapped. Outraged, she grabbed a chain she used to lock her bicycle and held it in a menacing way. "I'm not killing Jack over a busted jaw!" she shouted.

"Get her out of here!" someone yelled. "We're calling the cops!"

When all was finally calm, it was the hospital that had the change of heart. Years later Cuddyer had no deep regrets about the incident. "It worked," she would say. "They thought I was just some dumb little white kid."

Nowadays Nancy kept the peace. Her job was to keep Angell's waiting room running smoothly—move them in, move them out—a mission she made look easy. It certainly sounded simple enough: When clients arrived for an appointment, she sat them down on one of the benches. If it was an emergency, she scrawled the basics on the walk-in list and summoned a doctor, usually one of the interns. Then she hung a hand-sized blue plastic square with a white numeral on it—1 through 13—on a nail on the wall. This was so the interns, coming out of the examination rooms or from the innards of the hospital, could see how many emergencies they still needed to tackle. When the blue blocks read 1 or 2, Cuddyer's job was still simple enough. When the numbers got higher and the room filled and the *human* heart rates started climbing, Cuddyer truly earned her pay.

As with any emergency hospital, the interns handled the most life-threatening cases first. A walk-in usually required at least enough time to examine the animal, get a history, book it in if need be, and begin some sort of treatment.

The less urgent cases waited. These clients—their days dwindling, their pets still retching or coughing or licking at a laceration— inevitably grew restless. Usually, a loud sigh was the first sign of a storm rolling in. As the minutes sometimes stretched into hours, the sighs became strolls up to Cuddyer to ask just what the *hell* was going on.

"A boid!" a man grumbled one day as a newly arrived bird was allowed to see a doctor before his dog with a leg wound. "The boid's dead! It's on the bottom of its cage!"

The interns, meanwhile, with every new number, could practically feel their adrenal glands crunching down. Sometimes it was stressful enough just to come up with a diagnosis for the animal in front of them. At the same time, few could ignore a waiting room that was starting to look like Ringling Brothers and Barnum & Bailey. One look around, and you knew you were under the big top.

A breeder would appear one day with a cage full of adorable Newfoundland puppies, flopping over one another as they were wheeled in for cardiac tests.

A skinny, long-faced owner might resemble the greyhound at his side, while another man looked like his pug.

A family would leave an exam room, arms draped around one another, everyone sobbing, leaving behind their longtime pet, euthanized.

A girl would rush in—blood soaking her clothes, clutching her borzoi, with the skin ripped off its paw from the car that just hit it— then faint dead away.

A couple would be seen backing out of an exam room, video camera running, documenting their dog's visit. "Say good-bye!" one of them would say. "Bye! Bye!"

Indeed, every moment held the promise of intrigue, if not the outrageous.

Furthermore, people could talk with each other. Strangers had commonalities in their love of animals that crossed barriers of age, gender, race, and social status. Because it was their pets in for medical treatment and not themselves, conversation flowed more freely. Only in the Massachusetts penal system would someone be more likely to ask: "What are you in for?"

Friendships occasionally blossomed. Now and then an owner— sometimes demanding that Angell's staff keep his identity secret— would pay the bill for another who had fallen on hard times.

In terms of design, the area was as artful as an interrogation room. It consisted mainly of the counter Cuddyer sat behind and two long benches before her, also with gray Formica surfaces, less than ten yards across from each other. Most owners saw little more of the hospital than this and one of the nine examination rooms that ran to the right of Cuddyer's desk.

Visitors had a limited choice of reading material, usually MSPCA propaganda, a stack of dog-eared car magazines that some- one brought from home, and a day-old *Boston Globe.*

Someone in the organization was always talking about redeco- rating the waiting room, adding artwork, perhaps, or brighter colors. None of the customers, though, seemed to mind. After all, a spindly- legged Irish setter, its head resting across its master's feet, or an Angora cat, peeking from its carrier, was beauty aplenty. All the place really needed was a way to make sure the visitors—pets and people alike—got the service they wanted and, in the meantime, stayed under control.

Enter Nancy Cuddyer. She admonished mothers to restrain

their children, who might be touring the room, yanking a tail here and there.

She sweet-talked some anxious clients into returning to their seats and laid down the law for others.

She produced empty exam rooms when doctors had abandoned all hope.

She patiently explained to the woman with the gerbil in her hands that the greyhound she kept patting and calling "nice doggy" was actually bred to *chase* certain small, furry objects.

She separated warring canines and prevented untold other calamities.

She scurried back to the Hole, the intern office, and cajoled one or two interns who were off clinic duty—and swamped with their own work—into helping out. Occasionally, she just called them on the telephone. "There's a guy up here who thinks we're dickin' him around," she would say. "Do you think you could come up and see him for an exam and shots?"

In short, Nancy Cuddyer kept the lid on—usually. One day a longshoreman, fed up with waiting, threatened to sock her—and looked for a minute like he might.

Another time, Nancy herself lunged after a woman who had gotten too personal in her criticism. Coworkers restrained Cuddyer as some clients who had been watching the spectacle cheered Nancy on. "Hit her!" came one cry. "I'll hit her for ya!" offered someone else.

That day, Cuddyer was called onto Gus Thornton's carpet. "Well, Gus," she said, assuming her days at Angell were over, "is this it?"

"Nancy," he replied, "with friends like you, we don't need enemies."

And no, she wasn't being fired. Thornton was many things, but he was not insane.

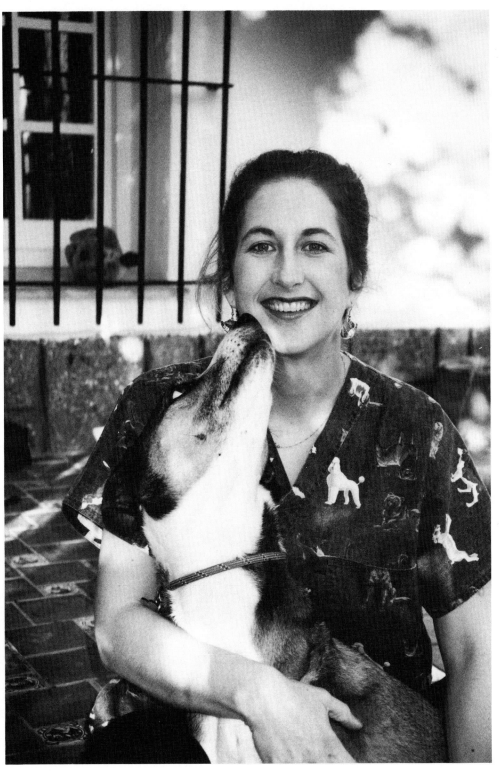
Lynne Morris, former veterinarian intern at Angell, and her dog Graham. *Photo courtesy of Eric P. Smith.*

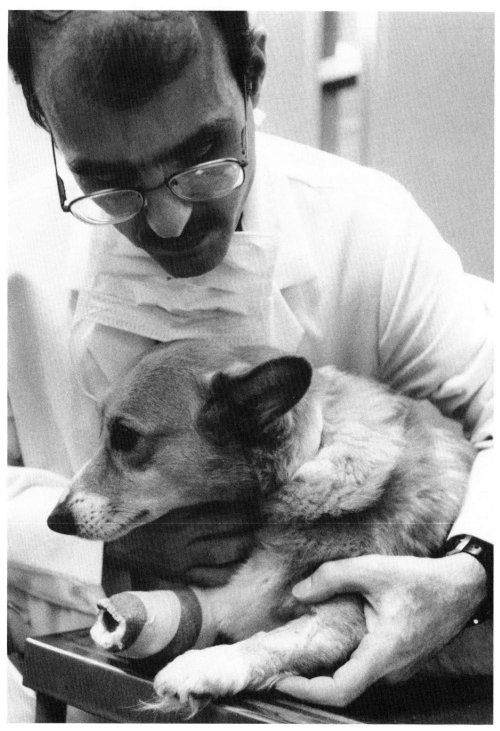

Paul Gambardella (Gamb), Angell Memorial Animal Hospital's chief of staff and orthopedic surgeon. *Photo courtesy of Steve Liss.*

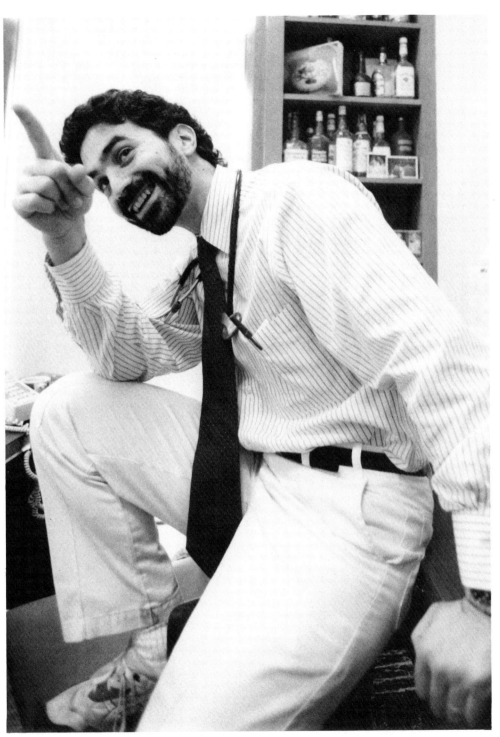

Doug Brum, Angell staff veterinarian and former director of the intern program. *Photo courtesy of Steve Liss.*

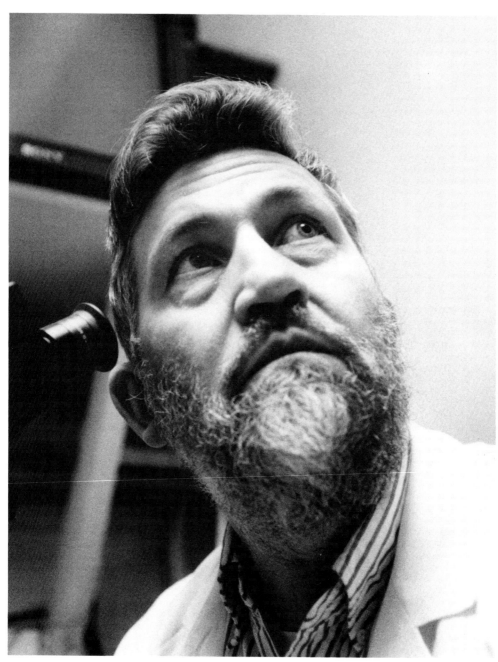

James Carpenter (Carp), former head of the department of pathology with more than thirty years of service at Angell Memorial Animal
Hospital. *Photo courtesy of Steve Liss.*

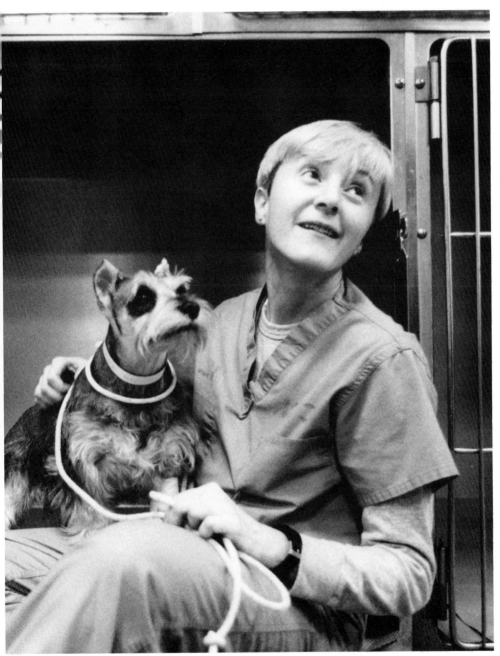

Joan Fontaine, ICU nurse at Angell. *Photo courtesy of Steve Liss.*

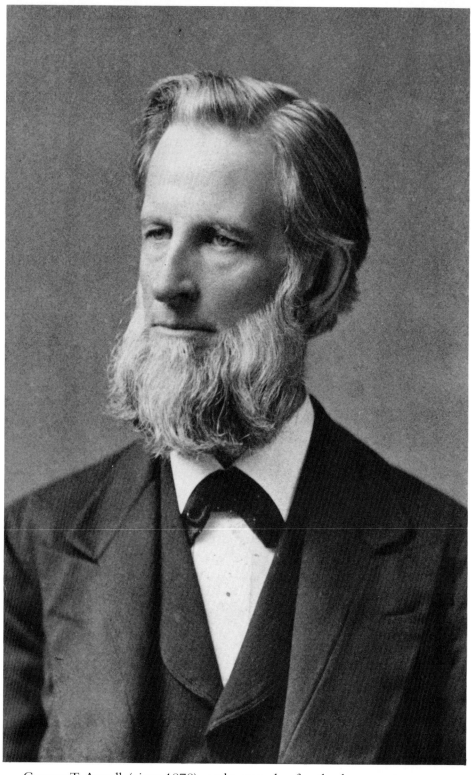

George T. Angell (circa 1878), early crusader for the humane treatment of animals. He founded the Massachusetts Society for the Prevention of Cruelty to Animals in 1868. *Photo courtesy of MSPCA.*

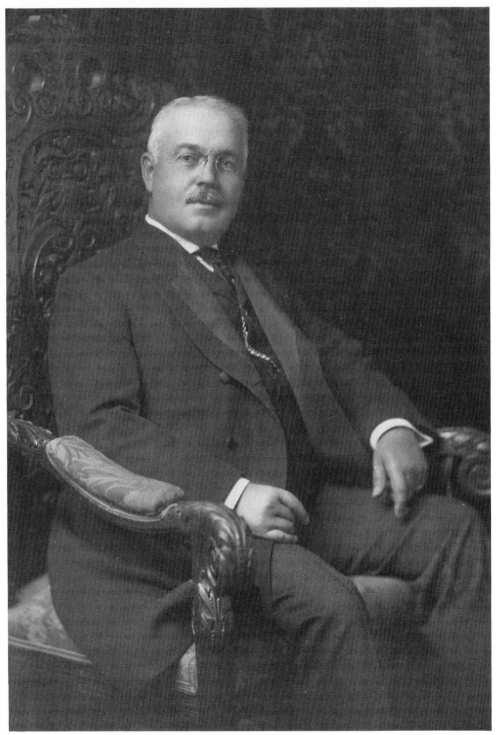

Francis H. Rowley (circa 1910), successor of George T. Angell as the president of the Massachusetts Society for the Prevention of Cruelty to Animals and founder of Angell Memorial Animal Hospital. *Photo courtesy of MSPCA.*

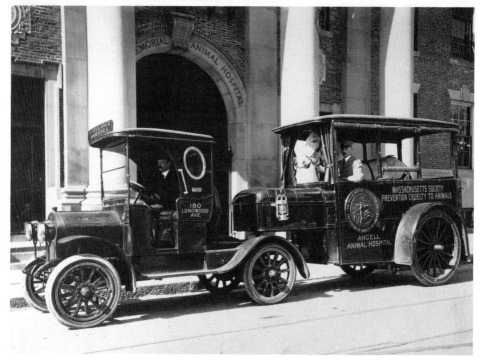

Angell Memorial Animal Hospital ambulance (circa 1917). *Photo courtesy of MSPCA.*

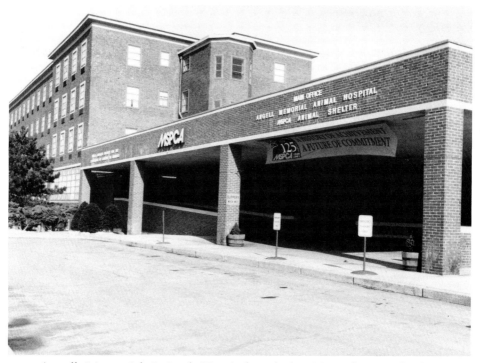

Angell Memorial Animal Hospital and the Massachusetts Society for the Prevention of Cruelty to Animals are housed in the same building. *Photo courtesy of Steve Liss.*

Backshop

INSIDE WAS ANOTHER ANGELL.

Beyond the examination rooms, a wide corridor on the first floor spanned the breadth of the facility. At one end was the intensive care unit; far off at the other, a set of doors led to the euthanasia room of the MSPCA's Boston shelter.

The hallway was a thoroughfare, with connections and exits to most everything within the hospital—the waiting room, surgery, cardiology, radiology. There were even rest stops—the lavatories and a cubbyhole where the surgery techs ate lunch. Practically everyone who worked in the hospital came this way sometime during the day.

Traffic was heaviest during rounds, when the surgeons and medicine staff met in their respective groups and subgroups to review the cases in the hospital. Sometimes as many as a dozen veterinarians, all in white coats and murmuring, would crowd down the hall, going from the wards, say, to radiology.

Late at night was a different picture. Only a skeleton staff was on duty, and most of the lights were extinguished. As a solitary intern stepped through the shadows, the hall seemed less like an interstate and more like a lonesome path through moonlit woods. The baying of a hound in the distance only added to the effect.

Not until dawn did the eeriness dissipate. The day-shift nurses showed up between seven and seven-thirty. Around that time, most of the interns and some staff doctors arrived to check their patients before rounds. The late-night intern, who worked until eleven or twelve the evening before, traditionally brought breakfast for the doctor who stayed all night. In the waiting room, owners delivered their dogs and cats for spay or neuter operations.

At eight, morning rounds began. So did the daily seminar for the residents down in pathology. In surgery the supervisors would soon be setting up equipment and planning the day's schedule. Calls increasingly trickled in to the receptionist, who invariably answered with a singsong "An-gell Memori-Al."

At first glance the place had the impersonal air of any medical setting. Sick people always seem dehumanized in a hospital, surrounded by aseptic conditions and medical gadgetry. Animals, being even closer to the natural world, look all the more displaced attached to an intravenous catheter or rolling down a hall on a gurney, tongues lolling out, anesthetized.

Fluorescent lights. Gleaming tile floors. Stainless steel. Few of Angell's surfaces were soft or inviting or comfortable. As you might expect, everything was designed with efficiency and cleanliness in mind. The result was a sense of coldness, and most staffers, preoccupied and pressured, did little to warm the atmosphere for outsiders or owners visiting their pets.

Yet even standing in the quiet desert, if one waits and watches, life reveals itself everywhere—small tracks in the sand, movement behind a rock.

At Angell the first signs of humanity were found in the soft-drink cans and the mugs of coffee sitting on the hallway floors, abandoned temporarily as staffers wandered into no-food-or-drink zones like intensive care and surgery.

Meanwhile, on the silver tinback that held a dog's medical records, someone had plastered a piece of white tape and scrawled special instructions: "Kiss often."

Most doctors had their names on their pagers, either written on medical tape or in raised letters on thin pieces of plastic; but one veterinarian attached a strip that identified him simply as "Boytoy."

Knickknacks the color of sugar cookies lined the outer window frame of the surgery suite where total hip replacements were performed. Molded from leftover acrylic "bone cement," the artwork included a serpent, a dolphin leaping through a hoop, and a hand in a defiant one-finger salute.

Not far from that was a posted memorandum from the director of surgery to housekeeping, pleading that something be done about a cockroach infestation: "HELP! Our situation is desperate.... We have found them in endotracheal tubes and syringes. One of our employees inadvertently took one home in her pocket."

IT WAS DIFFICULT TO DEFINE THE TWO HUNDRED or so people who worked at Angell Memorial Animal Hospital. Three-fourths were women; only one-eighth were minorities. They earned anywhere from $7.25 an hour as an entry-level ward attendant to well over $100,000 a year as a top-of-the-heap administrator or veterinarian.

They came from all backgrounds, from working class to affluent. Most of the lay staff hailed from around Boston, but the veterinarians, interns in particular, could be from anywhere in the country. Some staffers had grown up in the city; others on ranches. Some had degrees from Ivy League colleges; others just high school diplomas.

The overachievers were most evident on the veterinary staff; some spent most of their adult lives in college, vet school, and various training programs before ever having a true job. Even then, they would set aside family and personal obligations for a couple more years as they worked to become board certified in specialties.

Other employees were on their way somewhere. Some took low-paying jobs as attendants, technicians, or nurses to build their credentials for veterinary school or other careers involving animals. A number of Angell's nurses later worked as RNs.

Some of the personnel were exactly where they wanted to be, getting a regular paycheck, working with animals, and seeing something different every day. Many people made not only careers but lives out of Angell and the MSPCA. Some had started in the wards as teenagers, met their husbands or wives on the job, and stayed on until retirement.

Paulette Vartabedian had been a nurse for twelve years before the daily wear and tear led her to switch jobs and become the hospital's switchboard operator. She regarded each new day as an adventure, fielding calls about "rabbi shots" or how people could go about having their dogs "neutralized." One regular, an elderly inner-city black woman, often had questions about her cat, whom she identified as her "son," with language that sometimes got salty. Once she vowed to come by with an Uzi, at which point Vartabedian disconnected her. The woman poked speed-dial on her telephone and called right back to yell, "You damned honky bitch!"

Often callers asked Vartabedian for a diagnosis, or they sought advice. "My cat just fell five stories," they would say. "What should I do?" At other times she was the Miss Manners of animal welfare: "What's the most humane way to kill a lobster?" came one question.

"One of the most upsetting calls I got," Paulette said, "was a couple of years ago from a man who wanted to know how long it would take his cat to die if he hooked it up to the exhaust of his car. He didn't want the cat anymore, and he thought that was the humane way to do it."

Not everyone, of course, was content at Angell. A certain turbulence was simmering just below the surface. Someone was perpetually at odds with someone else. "One of the hallmarks of this hospital is that there's a lot of tension," explained intern Gary Block. "Everyone is constantly idling, waiting for a spark to go 'Kaboom!'"

The combatants and alliances changed from day to day. Sometimes it was management versus the lay staff's union, Service Employees Local 285. Sometimes it was the technicians or nurses feuding with members of the professional staff. Working at close quarters under stressful conditions could have virtually anyone snapping at someone else. "Everybody has their times when they hate working with each other," said ICU nurse Joan Fontaine, notorious herself for in-house squabbles. "It's bound to happen. Plus, we're all estro-synchronized, anyway."

The interns—low on the food chain, and newcomers to boot—had to guard against attacks from everywhere. During their first few months, as they learned the system and tried to build confidence, they were most vulnerable. One day it would be the nurses second-guessing their every decision, and the next a department head would rip all of them because a few missed a lecture. Some interns never seemed ruffled; others suffered from chronic battle fatigue.

What almost everyone shared, however, was a love for animals. Even if someone was assigned a battered desk in some lonesome corner of the hospital, inevitably a photograph of a dog or cat—often framed—would be found. Shots of the family were optional.

The secretaries, receptionists, and various other office workers had little reason to so much as pet a dog during their workdays, but most found a way. They would visit the shelter. They would sit by the entrance during their breaks, drinking in the passing parade. They would stop in the waiting room and greet a cute pet and its owner. Sometimes they knew the animal from previous stays. "Oh!" they would say to the accompanying human. "You're Fluffy's owner!"

When the subject shifted from pets to children, more than one staffer accidentally referred to a little tyke's parents as the "owners."

Not everyone, however, viewed animals the same way. Some veterinarians regarded their patients in the most clinical manner. Surgeons, for example, could often be seen standing over a dog or cat in the wards: "And this here is my total hip," one would say, seemingly denying the presence of a living creature, or "This is my acetabular fracture."

Every now and then a frustrated doctor or attendant crossed the line of decency and MSPCA standards, manhandling a resistant cat or dog. "Bruta-caine" is what the cynics called it. Some of the nurses told a story—perhaps apocryphal—about one veterinarian who was notorious for being rough with uncooperative pets. One day, they said, he slammed a cat to the exam room table to control it, then taped its hind feet together while he went to prepare to give it an injection. While the vet's back was turned, the cat is said to have crept down a table leg, dragged itself across the floor like a man dying of thirst, and sunk its teeth deep into the veterinarian's calf.

On the other hand, many employees were softhearted to a fault. Some spent half their workdays calling around to relatives and friends, looking for someone to adopt one animal or another before it was euthanized. Their own pets, meanwhile, were usually the ones no one else wanted, usually adopted from the shelter. So what if they were old or sick or missing a leg or an eye? One employee owned as many as eleven dogs at once, most of them rescued from euthanasia, before neighbors complained and the local dog officer was forced to act.

Many employees saw themselves as misfits out in the world, particularly when it came to animals. "I could never talk to anybody about animals the way I wanted to until I worked here," said Jennifer Snow, Doug Brum's liaison. "I went to a fair last weekend, and I asked my friend, 'Can I bring Roxanne?' And she said, 'No—why do you want to bring your *dog*?' I said, 'Well, *because*.' Now, if I'd been going with one of *these* guys, they would bring their dog."

Ward attendant Gerry Medeiros had been an Angell employee since 1967. She possessed a big heart for creatures of all kinds, largely because of the balm they have provided her. "I've always relied on animals," she said. "I read one time that somebody said, 'If animals could talk, we wouldn't love them as much,' because then they could reveal our innermost thoughts. We can cry to our animals. We can tell them our most deepest thoughts, and we know that we're safe. Even though the animal can't do anything for us to correct the problem, it releases that built-up pressure that we get inside of us. Many times I've cried over my dog's head."

Many people at Angell had friends who were bewildered at their despondency over their animals' deaths or illnesses. "It's just a cat," they would say. "You'll get another."

No one spoke that way at Angell. Instead, word whipped through the hospital when a staffer's dog or cat was in with a serious illness. It was as if a parent or spouse had taken sick. Sympathy came from all quarters. If someone was short of funds, even with the employee 50-percent discount, and management ordered that treatment be delayed, someone would take up a collection. And for days people would grouse about the organization's inhumanity to its own workers.

Money was hardly the reason most people worked here. Many were happy to find a job that involved animals. A few, in fact, never thought twice about stopping at an elderly woman's house on the way to work to make sure she was properly administering medication to her cat. And when a particular longtime patient showed up yet again, the attendants and nurses behaved like it was homecoming weekend. "Charley Johnson's back," they would say with a smile.

In the end, the infighting and complaints seemed the stuff of big families. In truth, there was a pride about working for Angell. Most who worked at the hospital saw themselves as being on the front lines of animal care.

To receptionist Vartabedian, those who worked at the hospital were different. She called them "Angellites." "Once an Angellite always an Angellite," she often said.

One retired surgeon liked to refer to those who worked at the hospital as Angells. Rose Henle, supervisor of sterile surgery, scoffed when she heard that nickname in reference to herself and her coworkers: "More like fallen angels, if you ask me."

12

The Battle

FOR ALL OF ANGELL MEMORIAL'S VETERINARY EX-
perts, medical gadgetry, and devotion to making sick animals well, the
truth was that miracles were rare. The hospital saw the toughest cases,
bar none. For a lot of animals, Angell was the last resort. Often the
battle was unwinnable from the word go. Always lurking was the
specter of financial considerations and the option of euthanasia.

The surgeons tended to have the best odds. Broken bones could
be pieced together, tumors excised, appendages amputated. Success or
failure was usually determined then and there, at the operating table.

The O.R. also provided a lot of definite answers. "You're standing in front of the radiology viewer," said surgeon Jim Boulay. "You've
got a radiologist, a medicine person, and a surgeon there. The radiologist is saying, 'It could be this, or it could be that.' The medicine person is like, 'We can do this, or we can do that.' And the surgeon's like,
'Let's just *cut* the damn thing. Let's just go in, open it up, and we'll find
out. If we're wrong, we're wrong.'"

Those in internal medicine, the Doug Brums, were willing to
accept less-immediate gratification, if any was to be had at all.

Sometimes the biggest success came in simply identifying what the actual problem was. (Jim Carpenter remembered one intern who dissolved in tears whenever she could not make a diagnosis.) With drugs, careful monitoring, and no small amount of customer hand-holding, animal lives were sometimes extended for six months, a year, or even a number of years.

Sometimes the best that could be hoped for was to keep the animal somewhat comfortable for a few more hours, maybe a day, so the owner had time to digest it all. One woman asked to take her old, dying cat out to watch the pigeons one last time. The cat probably got less from the experience than its owner, but it helped the woman cope. "You would like for the animal to have a nice peaceful demise," said veterinarian Jean Duddy, "but you also don't want to destroy a person in doing that."

Sometimes a client just needed a name to whatever disease was ravaging the pet before letting go was possible. Tests were run now and then that had little consequence on an animal's ultimate fate, but they went a long way in helping an owner find closure.

Certainly, all of the veterinarians had stacks of heartfelt thank-you letters from clients, oftentimes in the wake of their animals' deaths. There was hate mail, too, though. "I'll *never* bring another animal to you people again," read one. "*Never.* Not even an insect!!!" One intern received a picture of a little dog that had died on his watch; On the back the veterinarian was addressed as "murderer."

Recovery often came or went for reasons that actually had nothing to do with any treatment. Medical success or failure often turned on intangibles, even the unknowable. "That's why I got out of medicine," said Barbara Gores, a surgeon. "Pretty soon you're bringing out the holy water and the rosary and the feathers and bells."

In long-term cases, a veterinarian could not help but get to know the pet and its owner. When bad went to worse—sooner or later it always did—and the owner was falling apart, it was impossible to remain detached. Everyone agreed that if you stopped caring, it was time to quit, but how much of yourself could you give? "I find it runs in cycles," said Jean Duddy, "where you kind of bleed for everybody for a while, until there's just nothing left to bleed anymore."

Eventually, everyone ached for clients and their pets. Hardest hit were the interns, the hospital's veterinary field hands. Intent on saving the world, their emotional defenses still underdeveloped, and deluged with the most brutal cases, few of the young veterinarians came away unscarred. As often as not, animals came in dead or well on the way, leaving the interns with little more to do than say, "I'm sorry." Even an intern who'd gotten a handle on a problem would always worry how long their treatment would stave off the next crisis. Even when they finally got to sleep, many found themselves dreaming of the animals in their care.

Euthanasia, meanwhile, was both a blessing and a curse. It spared needless suffering. When animals were put down for financial reasons, however, it could weigh heavy on a caregiver's mind. "The euthanasia blues" was what intern Gary Block called it.

Sooner or later, almost every veterinarian had a good cry on behalf of a client and the pet. "I do cry a lot," admitted intern Nancy McCarron, who may have led her particular class in overall tears shed, "but then there are a lot of things that make you happy, too."

Nancy, age twenty-six, had fond memories of the middle-aged man from Dorchester who stormed in one afternoon with a stray cat that had been swung around in the jaws of a pit bull. The man, who had been outside gardening, scared the dog away and hurried the black-and-white cat into the hospital wrapped in a plaid shirt. The domestic shorthair, weighing all of six and a half pounds, was a wreck, its pelvis dislocated and fractured. Though the animal could be saved, as a stray its fate would probably be euthanasia, that is, until the fellow pulled out his credit card and asked McCarron whether an outdoor cat could become an indoor cat very easily.

All week McCarron had been swamped with PTSs, shorthand for animals that were, euphemistically, "put to sleep." She even had two women come in to have their dogs euthanized together. Most of her customers could hardly pay for the most basic services, but here was someone willing to go the distance for a stray. Nancy smiled.

A few days later, she called the man with an update. Surgery had been avoided. It looked like his new cat—identified as "No Name" on the records—was going to be all right and could go home in a day or so. "We *are* going to have to get this cat a name, though," McCarron said playfully.

"I already decided on a name," came the reply. "Nancy."

For many, the elderly were the toughest. Often they were deeply attached to their pets but were on a tight budget. The death of their dog or cat could be shattering. One older gentleman ended up with a bill close to ten thousand dollars for his aged poodle. One of the veterinarians was even overheard barking at chief of staff Gambardella, who had come by to discuss the mounting bill and the owner's refusal to euthanize his pet, "What do you want me to do, Paul? Put a gun to his head?"

When I spoke to the man, he said the dog had belonged to his late wife, for whom he still mourned six years after her death from cancer. For reasons that even he could not fully explain, he simply could not part with the animal. "I've got a lot of my wife's stuff at home yet," the widower said, "and I should just get rid of it and forget about the past. I've got her clothes. I've got drawers full of her stuff; I never got rid of it. Maybe it's the same with the dog; I don't know."

Cardiologist Neil Harpster, for his part, had built a large and loyal following of older patients and their geriatric pets, that he managed to keep alive long after other veterinarians had surrendered. Some people around Angell wondered whether Harpster even knew where the euthanasia solution was stored. As often as not, his clients were devastated when the end finally came.

"Generally speaking, in my experience it has been women that have been either unmarried or long term without a family, and their pet has become their primary companion," he said. "It's like losing a husband or a brother—that's what they feel has happened.

"I try to deal particularly carefully with people in that type of situation. I say, 'Now, the most important thing for you is to try to replace the pet. It won't be the same as the pet you had before, but it's really important that you get the companionship back again.'"

Make no mistake: a lot of sorrows washed up on Angell's shore. Still, the place saw plenty of victories, too. They were seldom turn-the-tide-heroics, though, as much as solid medicine, followed up with watchful nursing and a touch of grace from above.

Of course, there were the high-profile cases, the bullet-riddled or abused pet that Angell's staff nursed back to health. News reporters loved those stories, and they always got the hospital a lot of attention. But that was the stuff at which many on the staff half-sneered and privately rolled their eyes. If anything, the television cameras were a distraction, and on at least one occasion, a perturbed veterinarian read a TV crew the riot act.

What was the big deal, anyway? Around Angell, staffers knew that the best wins were the day-to-day wins, which was basically any time someone showed up to take an animal member of the family home. After all was said and done, even the victories that seemed easy meant the moon and stars to those involved.

One pensioner, for instance, brought in his eight-month-old German shepherd, who had been hit by a car and suffered a fractured femur. Clear and simple, the dog needed surgery, but the man lacked money for even an X ray. He thought maybe he should put the dog down.

Intern Will Johnson, who was handling the case, threw out an alternative from the old days of veterinary medicine. "Something you *can* try," he said, "is just to put him in a very close-confined space. Build him a box, and just take him out to urinate and defecate twice a day. Keep him very confined."

So the old man departed, and came back a week later with some money he scraped together for antibiotics. Johnson heard nothing from him for months. Finally, come spring, in they came again, the dog bouncing along like new. Johnson smiled. "Boy, I'm sure glad I listened to you!" said the client. "That was the best advice anybody ever gave me!"

Intern Gary Block, meanwhile, was baffled one evening by the Hispanic family who brought in their eight-pound Chihuahua that was stumbling over itself and seemed to be asleep on its feet. Block interrogated them and looked the dog over. He suspected neurologic damage—until he asked what the dog had consumed that night.

"Well, he just had a beer," someone answered, adding that the grandmother had thought the dog might like one.

Block's mouth dropped. "Do you mean to tell me that your dog just drank a beer?"

"Yeah, Doc. What do you think's going on?"

"What do I think's going on? I think your dog's drunk."

Block sent them home to let the dog sleep it off. He told them to keep an eye on him and bade them good night. Cheers, he said while chalking one up in the win column.

PART THREE *Working*

A person that started in to carry a cat home by the tail was gitting knowledge that was always going to be useful to him, and warn't ever going to grow dim or doubtful.

—MARK TWAIN, Tom Sawyer Abroad

13 Night

ANYONE WHOSE JOB IT WAS TO HELP HOLD A CITY together after dark—the cops, the paramedics, the emergency room physicians—knew about the night people: the folks who screamed of the CIA's "blue rays" seizing their minds, the binge drinkers, and the domestic disputees, to name just a few. After sunset they emerged in full force—the crazies, the raging, the desperate—exposing their pain, inflicting it on others, and disturbing what little order was left in the world.

Most late-night professionals looked to science for an explanation of such behavior. Thus, like the ancient Romans, they agreed that the full moon was to blame. If not *that,* the new moon. And if not that, all of the astronauts who had tromped around on the moon. So it was at Angell, where for half a century beginning veterinarians tended to the ailing pets of the Boston night.

So it was for Lynne Elizabeth Morris as she settled in one Wednesday evening in March. The winter had been tame. Today it was just a few degrees above freezing, but hardly a cloud marred the sky. Late that afternoon Lynne had wheeled into the hospital parking lot in her blue '81 Toyota Celica, with 180,000 miles on its odometer. She attended rounds, checked on her patients, and took an hour to exercise, in–line–skating with a fellow intern around nearby Jamaica Pond.

When Morris saw her first patient around five o'clock, the hospital had already begun its daily transformation. The office and support staff began to head home, followed in the ensuing hours by the staff veterinarians and, gradually, the interns. Although the waiting room was filling with after-work appointments and owners visited pets in intensive care, they too would soon depart. Before long all that remained would be the night supervisor, a few staff workers, two nurses in ICU, the overnight intern, who would be on round the clock, and Morris, who would stay until all of her cases were worked up, probably around two or three in the morning.

Like all of the interns, Lynne had been intimidated by the prospect of working nights—particularly overnight duty—with hardly anyone to turn to for help. She imagined the worst. Everyone, Morris figured, would now realize that she knew not a thing. She envisioned animals being hurt, even killed, their blood on her inexperienced hands.

When she first started, in fact, Morris went to Doug Brum to suggest that an on-call veterinarian be available every night, just in case an intern got in over his or her head. Nothing came of it, and by March Lynne had forgotten about it. When problems arose, she called Brum or one of the other doctors with whom she felt comfortable. If it was a particular vet's patient, she called that vet.

Still, she couldn't call for everything. Most decisions during those late hours were the intern's to make, and it would be a lie to say that no animals ever died because of an intern's failings. Paul Gambardella, for instance, once lost a spay patient when the ligature later slipped and the overnight intern failed to recognize that the animal was bleeding out.

A prayer that was engrained in Lynne's, and every intern's, psyche was that the cardiac and neurological patients, many with complicated and delicately balanced treatment plans, would rest easy until morning. When the heart monitor sounded or a pet had a seizure, Morris might find herself leafing madly through an emergency manual to help correct a problem.

No one—especially new veterinarians—could be expected to know everything. Thus, all the interns had moments when they calmly excused themselves from the exam room, ostensibly to take a call or check on another emergency, and then flung themselves down the hall to the library or the intern office to find a text to help.

Fatigue—some went as long as thirty-six hours without sleep—and a heavy workload were burdens every intern carried. As the year wore on, most were in a weary-stress state, which varied in intensity but never completely faded.

True, the internship had been modified in recent years to give the young doctors time to work normal hours for several weeks in surgery, for instance, or radiology. Still, even the most stoic among them worried about how fatigue and time constraints affected patient care.

Night. It was intimidating to be alone in the near-vacant hospital, especially for someone fresh out of veterinary school. In many ways, it added pressure. But in others, it diminished the stress and was liberating. No one was here to judge the interns, or second-guess them. At night it was ultimately their call. Not everyone liked that— some clients roared about neophytes handling their debilitated pets— but for the young veterinarians the decision-making experience was invaluable.

Now, as early evening embraced the hospital, Lynne Morris worked her way through a steady but relatively peaceful series of owners and their pets. By nine o'clock the pace quickened, and every case took on a sharp emotional edge. No surprise there: a new moon was overhead.

First came a pleasant, middle-aged couple with a white-faced, aging golden retriever that was panting endlessly. They brought along some chest X rays from a referring veterinarian but said he had given no indication of the dog's problem.

Lynne put the films up on the light box and looked the dog

over. "Your veterinarian didn't say anything about what might be wrong?" Morris asked evenly.

"Nothing."

Although it was hard to be certain for any given case, it was an old story. Any veterinarian could read an X ray well enough to know that this whiteness running across the chest and lungs on the shadowy films indicated fluid that most certainly did not belong there. Often, though, it was easier to point the client toward Angell and let someone else break the bad news.

It was too early to tell for sure, Morris said, but the odds were that something serious—maybe cancer—was raging inside. Now her voice was quavering, as it often did when she had to report the worst kinds of trouble. They could book the dog in for some tests, she continued, but the couple should know that the odds and financial considerations were probably not good. Fluid in the chest meant trouble, golden retrievers were prone to cancer, and this one was getting on in years.

One minute the couple had been laughing; now their eyes were brimmed red. Their previous dog had been euthanized here, and the thought of the same fate for this one was hard to take. They opted for the tests and left holding each other for support.

Next came a woman who was beside herself, quaking and talking nervously in disjointed sentences. Somehow or other, her dog had broken a nail, and it was bleeding. Morris stopped the flow in all of five minutes. She even bandaged the paw for good measure. But the woman was adamant that the animal be hospitalized. "I just got out of treatment," she said, "and I can't be worrying about this!"

She was followed by a bearded fellow who looked to be in his mid-thirties. He had been sitting impatiently, reading a book about computers, his cat in a crate at his side. The animal had already been in to have a broken leg repaired. He was here now, the man said, for an X ray and a cast change.

Morris explained that the radiologist was available only during the day. Lynne herself could X ray the leg, but it was better to have someone with more experience read the film. What's more, this was not an emergency, and it cost sixty dollars just to be seen at this hour. It would be better to return during the day.

Back and forth they went, the client growing more and more insistent. He was *sick* of the hospital, he said. Morris was the third doctor he had seen. "And they said I could come in for an X ray *anytime!*" he roared. Finally, Lynne surrendered. She took the cat and strode away toward radiology. "Jerk," she muttered to herself.

Later, after everything was done, the front office called to tell Morris that the client had just now taken his animal and stormed out—without paying. "If I knew it was going to cost this much," he had shouted, "I'd have put the cat to sleep!"

It was only fitting that around that time, in came Dynamite. At a hundred pounds, the rottweiler weighed only slightly less than Morris. But, he was only about half the weight of his owner, a beefy chunk of man with a face that would have been ideal over the steering wheel of a screaming tractor-trailer. They sat in the waiting room, a "Hogan's Heroes" rerun on the TV. The man, calmly waiting his turn, chatted and traded jokes with some owners across the room. A choke collar, with prongs that pinched the skin, encircled Dynamite's neck. Connected to that was his leash, a thick leather strap.

Lynne ushered them into an exam room. Dynamite had injured one of his front paws and it was becoming infected. While Lynne filled out some paperwork, the man kept talking to the dog. "Yeah," he said. "They're gonna give you the treatment." He laughed maniacally. "They're gonna give you the treatment, all right."

A low, throaty rumble emanated from Dynamite when Lynne went over. Without too much difficulty, she and the owner slipped a brown leather muzzle over his snout. A loose fit, she thought, but it should be all right. Morris crouched and barely touched the paw.

Instantly, Dynamite's muscled torso and skull, a bowling ball with snout and teeth, lunged at her in a guttural explosion of snarls and barks. Though the leather muzzle was still in place, the beast's jaws clacked wildly, his incisors all too visible from the opening in front.

Eyes wide, Morris dropped back on her hands, the dog leaning over her. The owner yanked the leash; Dynamite halted. Then the man laughed long and hard. "He's scared, more than anything," he said at last.

Morris, looking wan, arose and telephoned for an attendant to help restrain the dog. When the woman came, everyone took their places. Lynne tried once again to see the paw. Once again the animal burst forth savagely. Again the owner roared with mirth.

Morris shook her head in disbelief. "That's it," she said. "If you want, you can come back tomorrow and someone can sedate your dog. If you don't want to do that, I'll give you some antiseptic and some antibiotics, and you can see how that works. But he's not going to let me look at him tonight."

Resignedly, man and dog headed out. "You've got a ba-a-ad reputation," the owner told Dynamite. "A bad rep—a bad, bad rep."

They sat back down in the waiting room to wait for his wife. "Usually, I'll stop by Burger King, and I'll get him a hamburger after the vet's," I heard him tell another owner, "but not tonight."

He glanced at Dynamite sitting before him. "Nope," he said, "no hamburger for you tonight."

WHEN SHE WAS A GIRL, LYNNE MORRIS ALWAYS HAD animals prowling about her house. There was, of course, Mike, the family's collie-shepherd mix. Over the years there had also been chickens, a raccoon, fish, gerbils, and the garden-variety pet store turtles. Still, horses were her first love. She had been riding since the fourth grade.

Between that and having consumed all of James Herriot's adventures from the dales of Yorkshire, Lynne knew she would be a veterinarian. She expected to spend most of her time caring for horses and various farm animals, perhaps treating a few dogs and cats on the side. Her father, a retired carpenter, used to smile at the idea of Lynne's becoming a veterinarian, given how his little girl used to pass out at the sight of blood.

At the University of Maine in Orono, where Morris majored in animal sciences and minored in zoology, her outlook evolved. She took a strong interest in animal rights issues, abandoned red meat, and began to get a broader picture of veterinary medicine. It took her aback to learn how much of large-animal care revolved around animals as sources of income, be it in the beef industry or horse racing. Plus, veterinary care was so expensive that few owners, be they farmers or everyday equestrians, were able to take treatment very far.

"In large animals, it's much more of a money decision," Morris said. "A farmer might say, 'This cow is worth X dollars, so it's not worth it to me to do thirty dollars of blood work, because I'm going to lose my profit margin. And she's not a good cow, anyway, so we'll just ship her.'"

Like many who aspired to be veterinarians, Morris also saw that a career like Herriot's—caring for both large and small animals—was increasingly unrealistic in these fast-changing days of veterinary medicine. An onslaught of sophisticated equipment, new drugs, and the constant discovery of new diseases had irreversibly changed the field. There simply was too much to know about too many kinds of animals.

Small-animal medicine was already dividing into specialties and subspecialties. Going fast were the days when a veterinarian could do it all, from vaccinations to surgery and everything in between. As in human medicine, no one could know everything—and physicians had only one species to worry about.

When Morris attended Tufts's veterinary school, she was a classic example of the new breed of veterinary student. For one thing, she was a woman. Twenty years earlier, only a handful attended veterinary school; now it was well over 50 percent. Unlike veterinarians of previous generations, she embraced a philosophy that saw the intrinsic value and rights of all creatures. Morris ardently opposed the use of animals for experiments, for example, be it by students practicing surgical techniques or scientists seeking a cure for cancer. "Just because an animal isn't owned," Morris would say, "doesn't mean it has no value."

Veterinary schools have been slow to change their methods of training, long using unwanted dogs and cats to master surgical techniques. In recent years controversy has erupted on numerous campuses as veterinary students and professors advocating animal rights have challenged the status quo. Expulsions and lawsuits have made headlines at the University of California at Davis, the University of Pennsylvania, and Ohio State University, among other schools.

Not long after she arrived at Tufts, Morris and some classmates began discussing their opposition to the school's junior surgery lab. It was outrageous, the students said, to take healthy animals, operate on them, then euthanize them. Why use any living creature? Medical schools certainly never did.

Her sophomore year, Morris was among a dozen students who put together a proposal for an alternative lab in which the students could train on cadavers, then, supervised by surgeons at outside clinics, operate on animals that actually required surgery.

The school rejected it. The students were told that they would take the course as structured or not be allowed to go forward in the program. It was clear that their educations and careers were on the line.

"We said, 'Fine—kick us out,' and they didn't," Morris said. "We had enough people that we knew that wouldn't happen. Senior year, they rely on you quite a bit to staff the hospital, especially the large animal unit. We knew that if they kicked us out, they wouldn't have the bodies to take care of the hospital."

Pressured, the administration devised its own alternative, having Morris and the others work on cadavers in surgery lab and then put in extra time assisting in the hospital's surgery department.

"It was an idea whose time had come," Morris said, "and I'm sure they were a little scared. We hadn't gone to the newspapers, but if we did, you could just see *The Boston Herald*: 'Vet Students Forced to Kill Dogs.' We would have done that."

One adage has it that the top third of any veterinary school graduating class ends up becoming the best researchers. The middle third goes on to become the best practicing veterinarians. And the bottom third—well, they go on to make the most money. Morris graduated in 1990, smack in the middle of her class. She came away with her veterinary school degree and a debt the size of a small mortgage.

After graduation dozens of internships were available, but Morris applied for only one—Angell. When the dust of the nation-wide computerized matching program had settled, she found herself out in the cold. She entered the match again a year later. Rejected by Angell once, she now ranked the Animal Medical Center in New York as her first choice. The Boston animal hospital was now a distant second; they had their chance, Morris told herself.

Fate, however, gave both a second opportunity. This time the match landed her at Angell. Of course, she accepted.

EMERGENCY WORK FRIGHTENED SOME INTERNS. IT was especially scary in their first months at Angell, when they felt like outsiders and they were just awakening to their talents, or lack there-of, as working veterinarians. In the maelstrom that a crashing pet often brought, some interns looked for whatever security they could find. Many turned to cookbook medicine, treating every animal that had been mangled by a car, for instance, with a somewhat standard amount of fluids and steroids, instead of properly assessing each crisis individually.

Some interns thought they knew more than they actually did. Fueled by immaturity and ego, they plunged into their cases with the abandon of invasionary paratroopers. They refused to ask for help. No procedure daunted them. And it never took long for staff members and nurses to identify the worst offenders and to try, with varying degrees of success, to rein them in.

Lynne Morris liked critical care. And the staff considered her good at it. Among other things, she could think on her feet and set priorities in the midst of a storm. She learned that if she had five clients waiting, it was unnecessary to immediately suture, for instance, an animal's lacerated leg. She could book it in, wrap the injury, and return to it when calm settled again. (Battlefield conditions make it less simple than it may sound.)

Like any intern, Morris also had her off days. Once she was helping to ultrasound a dog with cancer, when suddenly its heartbeat fell weak and off rhythm. Morris raced the animal to intensive care and prepared to use the defibrillator to jump-start the creature's heart back to a normal pace. "All clear!" she yelled, then pressed the baby-sized pads against the animal's chest.

Suddenly, she felt a rush of electricity surge through her body. Having never used the equipment, Morris assumed that such a treat was normal. She shocked the dog again, but this time she herself felt nothing. "Oh, no!" she said as it dawned upon her. "I think I defib-rillated myself" the first time.

At times Lynne hesitated to perform a procedure, such as a spinal tap, that she had never tried. Yet it was not so much fear as a need to get it straight in her mind, of knowing exactly what to do. That was what the staff wanted in the interns—respect for the potential consequences of their work, not fear, and certainly not impudence.

One intern rite of passage came when an animal had excess air in the chest and required a chest tube. The goal was to use the palm of the hand to drive a trocar up between the animal's ribs and into the chest. When this was executed properly, the sharp-tipped stylet was then pulled out, and the air flowed from the tubing that remained. When performed wrong—and even Angell's finest had their disasters—fatal injuries, including skewering the heart, could result.

On her first case, a dog, Morris did her job almost perfectly. Her second one, a few days after Dynamite's appearance, was a domestic shorthair cat named Maggie that had a pyrothorax, pus in the chest. With Alicia Faggella and Doug Brum on hand that afternoon, Lynne solidly struck the trocar; a moment later the cardiac monitor fell into the high-pitched hum that for all real purposes said "Endgame." All attempts at resuscitation—including Morris's slicing open the animal and massaging the heart—failed.

Lynne was sobbing by the time she finally gave up; she felt certain she had punctured Maggie's heart. Yet no blood had run back up the tube, as it surely would have if she had hit an aortic vessel. When Faggella and Brum poked their gloved fingers around inside the animal's chest, they were surprised to find she had thick pockets of fibrous, vascularized tissue. Morris apparently had pierced one of them, causing the cat to bleed out.

Ten minutes later Lynne got word that Maggie's owner wished to have the body returned for burial. Sad-faced and quiet, she set about suturing the incision and wrapping the cat's midsection to avoid shocking the woman. Just as Morris was finishing, intern Beth Campbell came by. "You know," Lynne said tiredly, "I go by this funeral home every day. And I always say to myself that I could never be a mortician. Yuck—preparing dead bodies. Now look at me."

Campbell pondered that for a moment and patted her friend on the back. "Well, at least you don't have to put lipstick on her."

LIKE THE DOG DYNAMITE, OVERNIGHT DUTY HAD A bad rep. Not every night was lunacy. Sometimes business was so slow that Morris would mount the stairs to a small bedroom upstairs as early as midnight and sleep until dawn. Otherwise, she could catch up on her patients already in the hospital, or on her paperwork.

Night was a good time, too, to reflect. During the day Angell was constantly abuzz with people and animals, churning like a giant machine, relentlessly demanding. Come dark, and you could finally turn off a bit. It was easier, too, to hear yourself think.

Early one morning, the clinic stagnant, we sat in the intern Hole, talking about her plans. Lynne was at her desk, which was in a corner, wedged against a refrigerator and decorated with pictures of her pets, fiancé Eric, and friends.

She said she sometimes wondered about the veterinarians at Angell. So many were such hard chargers. From the time they were children, some small piece of them was always focused on this work. It gathered momentum come high school and propelled them through college, veterinary school, internships, residencies, and board certification exams. One former Angell intern was such an over-achiever that he eventually decided to scrap veterinary medicine and go back to school—medical school.

For herself, Lynne wasn't sure she wanted to keep charging. She had just turned twenty-eight. She had no burning desire to go on and become a surgeon, say, or an oncologist. Internal medicine interested her, but the trade-off in time to become a specialist was more than she wanted right now.

Some of Angell's veterinarians urged Gambardella to hire her, but Morris had other plans. After she got married in August, she was moving to North Carolina, where Eric was stationed, for a year. She hoped to find a temporary job at a veterinary clinic. She wanted time to enjoy her husband and her two mongrels, Leah and Graham, and she longed for a garden to dig around in.

Beyond that, who knew? Sometimes she remembered the flower shop her mother used to own, its pleasant fragrance, and what a happy place it had been. Sometimes she considered the Peace Corps. She and Eric had discussed adopting wild horses out West.

Few things had made Morris or her family prouder than when she finally became a veterinarian. It had put her in debt to the tune of $60,000, it was wearying, and it had cost precious time that could have gone to family and friends. These days, though, Lynne looked around and saw a lot of people who were wretched in all kinds of jobs and, worse, had no idea of what would save them. "For me, I *know* that this is what I want to do and this will be my career," she said. "I'm just happy that I know. No matter what, I have this degree, and nothing is going to take that away. What I decide to do within veterinary medicine, that's not important right now. It's just important that I have this degree and I can use it."

Morris had worked hard to get to this point. At the same time, she wanted room for her life. She looked around at Angell's staff, which included some of the best veterinarians anywhere, and wondered: "It's weird: all these people here keep striving and striving. It's like it never stops. Everyone's trying to get somewhere. The other day I was thinking about who's happy here and who's not happy here—"

"Who's not happy here?" I cut in, ever hungry for gossip.

"Well," Morris replied, refusing to bite, "let's just say that Doug Brum is one of the ones who's happy."

14
Dr. Feelgood

IN JUST A FEW DAYS, RITA MOORE AND HER ANCIENT, gray miniature poodle, Myra, had become well known to Nancy Cuddyer and the front office staff. At first glance the woman seemed ordinary enough. She was thirtyish, petite, with straight black hair. Her clothes were well worn but clean and neat. That characterization applied to her person as well. She seemed weather-beaten, yet she maintained a certain dignity of appearance. She materialized one spring day embracing the dog, which, unknown to her, was dying.

Myra was one of Doug Brum's patients. He had inherited the animal—and Moore—four years earlier, when as a favor he handled some cases for Mike Bernstein, head of internal medicine. Since then, whenever Moore appeared at Angell, Bernstein would wave his hand in dismissal. "Brum's client," he told the liaisons. "That's Brum's client now."

For his part, Doug took pleasure in the customers and cases that everyone else avoided. He had always been that way. Back when he was in veterinary school, working during the summers for his veterinarian cousin, he would always enthusiastically volunteer for some of the vilest jobs, whatever no one else wanted to do, and pretend he liked it. It won him some strange looks and, in the end, a lot of appreciation. What's more, he found that once he got going, there was a lot of personal reward in the work itself.

So was there in having Moore as a client. Brum never felt his boss had dumped her on him, not even when it became clear that she was mentally tortured and that sweet Myra was probably her last link to reality. Brum figured she was better suited to his temperament than Bernie's, anyway.

Try as he might, though, Doug's current efforts to learn about Myra's latest condition were disheartening. "Was the dog coughing?" he asked the owner. Yes. Was the dog sneezing? Yes, also. Yes, in fact, to pretty much everything. That was not all: Moore wanted to add that her landlord had poisoned the dog recently. Then she murmured something about a rapist. Also, she had given the dog meat juice the other day, which might be the problem. And she had accidentally stepped on her paw.

Thus enlightened, Doug set to examining the dog and noted that she kept licking around her mouth. When he peered deep into her throat, he discovered a tumor that ran from the tonsils on down the esophagus. To complicate matters, tests showed the dog to be in renal failure. Adding to her misery, Myra was septic: a deadly infection was running rampant through her bloodstream. Any one of the ailments could be the death of the creature. Though probably not long for this earth, the little dog was in fact retaining her place among the living.

Brum deemed the case an emergency; even though Moore had little money, Myra was admitted. The dog was stabilized, and a surgeon resected part of the malignancy. It was impossible to remove it all without causing serious harm.

Myra was housed in intensive care, and as the bill inched toward a thousand dollars, Brum could do little for the animal beyond keep her alive day by day. Financial office staffers, meanwhile, repeatedly took Brum aside, questioning him: How long would this animal remain in the hospital? What was her chance of ever recovering?

Couldn't he talk to the owner about euthanasia? The bill was climbing, and though financial assistance was available to the poor, the hospital was reluctant to let bills spiral ever upward for cases that were hopeless.

Doug nodded that he understood, but then shrugged. He had tried on several occasions to speak to Moore about euthanizing the dog—out of mercy more than anything else. The animal seemed not to be in deep pain, true, but pure and simple, she was dying. Any quality of life she once had was gone. Anyone could see it. Moore, however, adamantly rejected the suggestion.

"One of the hardest things about being a veterinarian is that sometimes you know or think that an animal should be put to sleep and the owner won't let you do it," Brum told me at one point. "To me, that's the worst—the worst."

He related an anecdote about a woman who once instructed him to go to any lengths to save her aged, obese, and dying German shepherd rather than euthanize it. Ravaged with a variety of diseases, the dog lost circulation to one leg, which became gangrenous. Though the dog could never stand on three legs because of its weight, the owner could not bear to part with it. Unable to change the woman's thinking, Brum instructed the surgeons to amputate. Soon after, another leg began to go, and again the woman said no to euthanasia. She even threatened suicide if the dog died.

"Just imagine," Brum recalled. "The nurses had to lift this dog four times a day and turn it on its other side and care for the sores it was getting on its body. The dog was urinating and defecating all over itself. It wouldn't eat. It was about this time that I started talking to the woman's psychiatrist. We were getting ready to amputate the other leg; thank God the dog finally died." The owner did not kill herself, for which Brum was grateful, but the case made him forever wary.

Moore never said she would take her own life. She captured Brum's attention—and sat Cuddyer bolt upright—when she would appear all of a sudden in the lobby or crowded waiting room and shriek, "Save my dog! You must save my dog!"

Moore had no phone and usually showed up unannounced. So it was that Brum, invariably in a meeting or tending to other clients, learned of her arrival from Nancy Cuddyer's matter-of-fact pages: Rita Moore is here to see you.

Now and then, Moore would impulsively call from a pay phone. When Doug arrived for work one morning, he found among his telephone messages a note scrawled at five in the morning by the overnight supervisor: "Rita Moore called, thinks her pet was poisoned by a local rapist—her landlord. Wants dog police to investigate. Also wants X rays of pet's head, neck, and chest."

For all her efforts, Moore was but one of the stressors eroding Brum's spirits. Gambardella was pressing him for progress on developing the Wellness Program. A new class of interns, for which Doug was responsible, was less than a month away. The current class, most of whom he considered friends, was soon departing. And, all at once, it seemed, springtime had brought a boom in business: annual vaccinations, heartworm tests, hit by cars, and, for reasons known only to the heavens, a run on animals to be euthanized. All this in addition to Brum's typical cavalcade of chronically ill patients and their owners.

These days Doug found Angell cutting deeper into his evenings. He would leave for home at nine o'clock, ten. It felt like being an intern again—only now he was director of the intern program —as he bounced from patient to patient, sometimes a dozen or more animals under his care at once. In one heart-wrenching day, he euthanized six pets. Among them was a dog belonging to a staff member and friend, an animal he had been treating for some time. That case, and the touch-and-go chemotherapy on another Angell worker's pet, had left Brum emotionally depleted, or as he put it, "sizzled."

These situations brought him knee-deep into the pain of his coworkers and friends, making it impossible to psychologically shield himself, and wore away at his psyche. "Sappers" is what one colleague called such cases. "I think I've cried more in the last two days than I've cried in years," Doug said. "I feel like quitting." He could feel the pressure grow around the sockets of his eyes.

Breaking bad news, though a fact of life in his line of work, was not Doug's forte—at least in some people's minds. Some staffers preferred to take their ailing pets to veterinarians who internalized less and, in the parlance of an old movie, gave it to them straight. "He just loves people," explained Jennifer Snow, Brum's liaison. "He hates to see people hurt. When my parents brought their dog in to see Doug, and she wasn't doing well, what he told them in the exam room and what he told me on the way down to draw some blood were two different things. And I had to tell my parents. He said, 'Well, Jen, I didn't know them well enough.' I said, 'Do you know *any* of your clients well enough?'"

At home these days, Brum was less than pleasant company for Sue. When Brum finally got home, he did little more than eat, stare vacantly at the television, and sag into bed. "If I worked like this all the time," he said, "I would have to leave Angell. It's something I promised Sue, especially if we have kids. My family is going to be my priority, so this has to change."

Sometimes Brum toyed with dropping out completely and becoming a high school science teacher or an astronomer. When business got like this, a lot of other professions shined bright.

It was during this stretch that Doug began to dream about Angell. One night he envisioned coming into work and finding dozens and dozens of telephone messages—more than anyone could ever field—awaiting him. "I was so depressed, and I felt so beaten," he recalled, "so when I woke up, I was happy. So what do I do? I come into work, and there's a huge pile of messages."

One night it was almost midnight before he finished. Rather than drive home, he went to a convenience store for a TV dinner, devoured it back at Angell, then dropped away to sleep, only to resume at five the next morning.

During the most difficult days of his internship a few years earlier, Brum had fed off the energy and fellowship of his intern mates. Although he was now a mentor to the young doctors, he still took comfort in their company. "Spiritual fortitude," he called it.

Brum invited the interns into his office for conversation and shots of bourbon. During his own internship, Doug and some fellow

interns, along with off-duty nurses and others, had held some outrageous after-hours parties back behind the scenes. There had been
dancing and enough alcohol consumption to float them out to sea.
Those impromptu celebrations eased the pressure and unified the
interns. Like a veteran of war, Brum treasured those days of height-
ened sensitivities.

As he marched toward his mid-thirties, Doug was leaving
debauchery behind. Sometimes, though, when his workload got hellish and his responsibilities at home increased, he cut a melancholy figure; he seemed to long for that old spirit and sought to recapture it,
if only momentarily.

This intern class, however, largely leaned toward pizza and soft
drinks. Some of them, of course, enjoyed a stiff drink and merrily
took part in Brum's rituals. Others agreed out of politeness. Lynne
Morris, for one, treasured Brum as a colleague and a friend, but she
had to admit that when she raised her glass and tipped back a drink,
it was less because she needed it and more because Doug, who looked
so sad, needed a friend.

RITA MOORE SAT ON THE CURB OUT BY THE GUARD
booth and the forbidding brick wall that marked the entrance to
Angell Memorial. Clad in a gray sports coat and bright green pants,
she hunched over her Bible, absorbed in Leviticus.

Brum stepped from the shadows of the building's overhang and
into the hard sun of a Tuesday afternoon. Some colleagues had been
good-naturedly jibing him about his unenviable client—by now,
notorious for her waiting room demonstrations—and his willingness
to attend to her curbside. Brum smiled, but the entire matter was
gnawing at him as he walked down the driveway toward her. How
could he make her understand? What could be the resolution of
Myra's case?

Traffic growled and rattled by. Some cars rolled into the lot, a
dog here and there peering from the passenger window. Brum greeted Moore and squatted like a baseball catcher. He summarized Myra's

condition. Moore seemed to pay attention. The kidneys seemed slightly better, Brum said, and the septicemia was somewhat improved, also, but they were not out of danger. The remaining cancer was inoperable; the dog was dying, he said.

"You treat," Moore insisted. "You treat my dog, Doctor."

"I don't think so," Brum said somberly.

Now she was crying. "I did this; I did this to my dog. I waited too long, too long to treat. I squeeze too tight. I didn't give the pills on time."

"No! Stop it! Stop!" Brum made a striking motion, as if speaking to someone deaf. "You can't keep hitting yourself. Stop beating yourself up!" He paused for a moment. "Do you know what causes cancer?"

After a moment, she uttered a quiet "No."

"No. None of us do. It's the food. It's the air. We don't know. If we knew, we'd win the Nobel Prize."

"Treat—can't you treat cancer?"

"No, not this cancer. Maybe at one point, but not all of it, and not now. What we have to do is decide what to do next."

Euthanasia, however, was out of the question to Moore, and medically not much was left for Brum to do. The dog would leave intensive care in a day or two, he told her, then be transferred to the general wards. She could probably take Myra home Saturday, though it wasn't the solution he thought best.

He gave Moore a sad good bye and started back up the incline of the driveway, quiet at first, then wondering aloud whether he had been too hard on her. He was angry at himself because nothing he said had really registered. "You know what the worst part of this is? The worst part is that *I'm* going to have to sit here and watch this dog slowly die."

He was back inside for five minutes, talking to a staff member near the front desk, when a building supervisor stepped over. "Hey, Dr. Brum," he said, "that girl you were with—is she OK?"

Brum looked over. "Why?"

"Well, she's out there laying on the grass crying. What is she, some kind of nut?"

Soon after, when Doug was home, his wife told him it was time to stop. He simply couldn't keep running outside to console this woman, getting so involved. He was already emotionally drained from overwork, and this was not helping matters.

"It's been four times you've gone out there for Mrs. Moore," she said. "She needs help, yes, but not from *you*. She needs professional help."

That Saturday Moore brought Myra home. On Tuesday the dog was back, obviously dying. That evening she succumbed.

It took a couple of days before Brum, relieved for Myra's sake as well as his own, could get word to Moore. When he finally did, Doug sensed that she took it well. She cried some and blamed herself, but she seemed to have understood death was coming. Then she drifted off, back into the city's faceless populace, more alone than ever. Doug Brum went back to work.

15

The Cutting Room

THE DOG, A FIVE-MONTH-OLD RETRIEVER MIX, WAS named Goldie. Nine days earlier he had been trounced by a car. Fate spared his life but not his left hind leg. The thighbone had shattered in such an ugly, jagged fashion that all who even glanced at the subsequent X rays wound up dropping open their mouths and staring in horror.

By the time Goldie reached Angell, he had already logged substantial time on the operating table. The original veterinarian, a private practitioner in Cambridge, had first tried to mend the bone, shattered just above the knee, with pins. When it was obvious, a few days later, that failure was imminent, he removed the pins and opted for a splint. When that seemed futile as well, he started to worry and referred the owner to Paul Gambardella.

The third surgery in Goldie's young life was scheduled for a gray Friday afternoon. It was just after lunch when the animal was anesthetized, prepped, and wheeled into sterile surgery. Inside were six surgical suites, open-ended stalls separated by concrete, windowed walls. The operating room technicians, bored by the drab decor and dreaming of more exotic ports, had taped signs in each suite, designating them "Cancun," "Japan," "Munich," and the like. Usually, at least one radio was on, though sometimes as many as three were going at once. Today a soft rock selection, Gambardella's favorite, was wafting through the unit.

In Cancun, suite four, the chief of staff summoned one of the three techs, whose duties included tracking down surgical instruments and taking care of whatever other needs arose: "Mary Lou, I think you'll have to get me some toys here." Cloaked in blue, the chief of staff rattled off the hardware he needed to hold open the surgical cavity and to keep the bones in place while he operated. "A couple Gelpies, a large Lane, small reduction forceps."

An intern named Julie Thorndyke was his assistant. "My main objective here is stability—alignment and stability," Gambardella told her. He then pointed to the two radiographs on the light box against the wall. "But I think I'm going to have a hell of a time achieving that because of that split."

For Gambardella, it was nice to be back in the O.R., complicated fracture and all. It bothered him that the demands of a seven-million-dollar budget and unhappy clients kept him away more often than he'd like. "I'm slipping," he said one day, worried. "I'm not doing anywhere near the surgery I did a year ago. Another year or two, and I'm gonna be far enough behind, behind in being in the thick of it, that I may have to stop entirely.

"You don't lose your manipulative skills. When I go to the operating room and make an incision, even if I haven't done it in a month, it all comes back. But what I'm losing is the fine tuning and the advancement. I try to read my journals, but then in order for you really to take that new information and learn it and know it, you've got to put it to use. That's what makes you a better surgeon and keeps you on the cutting edge of surgery. I'm not doing enough numbers."

When he did make it to the O.R., Gambardella was a happy

man. For the techs, he was always easy to take. Some of the surgeons had tempers, and now and then, when everything was going to hell at the operating table, they would verbally assault the hired help. On occasion an instrument slammed to the floor or against a wall. One agitated surgeon heedlessly heaved a fracture-repairing pin across the room and pierced a tech in the thigh.

Gambardella, of course, had his frustrating moments, too. When he was younger, he could hardly contain himself watching an intern or resident endlessly struggling with a procedure that he himself could finish in a fraction of the time. An intern could take two hours to get through a spay; at his peak Gambardella took but six minutes.

Though rare, Paul, too, was known to flare up during an operation. "One time he had an acetabular fracture that wasn't going well," remembered fellow surgeon Jim Boulay, "and he was pissing up a storm." However, a tech sometimes noticed the chief of staff quietly singing to himself when he came upon a knotty problem during an operation. Just thinking of it made her laugh. "Maybe he's happier when he's stressed," she said.

The biggest complaint the techs could muster about Gambardella was that he talked too much: hockey-playing sons, Boston Celtics, a veterinary junket to Germany. Periodically, one tech joked, she had to remind him that he did have surgery to perform.

Now the chief of staff and the intern stepped over to the silvery operating table where Goldie lay, an anesthesia tube in his slackened mouth, his body covered with aqua-colored drapes. Nothing was exposed but his shaved hind leg, now a rich yellow from having been swabbed with antiseptic.

Gambardella fingered the scalpel and began to slice into the thigh, cutting through skin and muscle until bone was revealed. The plan was to attach a titanium plate to the broken parts, fortifying the injury until what Gambardella called the "old folks"—Mother Nature and Father Time—returned the bone to strength.

Once he actually surveyed the damage, Gambardella knew his fears were well-founded. The destruction had been so severe, so much the opposite of a clean break, that the two basic pieces of bone barely touched, let alone fit together, when Gambardella tried to unite them. Some of the bone had simply been shattered to bits, leaving a gap at the point of the break and threatening stabilization and, in turn, any chance of healing. Matters were only complicated by the dog's youth. Puppyish buoyancy would make it difficult to keep him off the leg.

Paul sniffled under his mask, enduring a cold, and ran his gloved finger along the break, then slid it underneath. "This," he said quietly to Thorndyke, "is really a mess." The misaligned bones had already begun to ossify, requiring Gambardella to chisel away at their surfaces so as to smooth them. To have any hope of keeping the parts properly together, he would trim a quarter of an inch from the lower section, which would shorten Goldie's leg and slightly affect his gait.

Being an orthopedic surgeon was an ideal job for Gambardella. At the same time, it sometimes revealed by comparison how uncomfortable he felt dealing with the amorphous problems of the chief of staff's office. "The way my mind works," he said one day, "is that I have to reduce everything down to simple parts and then fix it. You can't do that with everything, and that's what frustrates me. I find having loose ends difficult to tolerate. When an individual is disgruntled, it bothers me. If there's a program we're getting off the ground, it eats away at me until I see how it's gonna go.

"In order for me to feel comfortable, I've got to see all the parts. What makes me happy is to see that all those parts are fitting well. If something's broken, we fix it. We work, work, work until it's fixed."

So it would go today. Goldie's surgery took nearly two hours. A bone graft from the ilium had been required to fill the gap, and the plate did not attach easily. On and on the operation went.

At one point, a fire alarm sounded. Since an intern's pet dog had recently jumped up and sounded the alarm, everyone today assumed this was another false warning—only a tech announced, "This one's for real!" She said she saw firemen rushing through the halls in full gear, making for the boiler room. The alarm—a horn that bleated and whooped—shook the building for almost fifteen minutes before it was silenced and declared to have been sounded in error. Yet neither Gambardella nor anyone else in surgery had budged. "I don't care if the place is burning down," Paul had muttered into his mask. "Just stop that infernal noise!"

One of the aspects Gambardella always liked about surgery, in fact, was that it required his undivided attention. No one could tap him on the shoulder here and expect very much in return. His schedule book remained in his coat pocket, hung on the wall in dirty surgery. Telephone calls had to wait. Even bomb threats, which Angell had experienced once or twice, failed to move him.

Gambardella looked worn as he stepped back to inspect his handiwork before closing up the leg and sending Goldie off for post-op radiographs. It was less than an ideal repair job, he thought, but it was the best he could do; the dog should heal. Gambardella would know better when he saw the new films and when Goldie came back in a week or two.

Dave Knapp, a surgeon in his early thirties, having finished with his own project in the next suite, ambled over. For a minute or two, he quietly surveyed Paul's finished product and nodded in approval.

Then his eyes wrinkled in a smile above his surgical mask as he leaned in toward the intern. "Ask him," Knapp said in a stage whisper, "if the toes are supposed to be pointing backwards like that."

16

Vivos Docent

A COUPLE YEARS BACK, JIM CARPENTER COMMITTED a serious blunder.

Doug Brum had sent down a sample from a cat he had examined, and pathologist Carpenter reported back that the animal had cancer. As a result, Brum's clients chose to euthanize their pet.

The problem came when the cat was slit open for an autopsy and Carpenter went to compare what he had seen in his microscope to the actual tumor. "I'm telling you," he would later say, "I did the best job of an autopsy that could be done in the world. Why? *Because I wanted to find tumor!* But I didn't find tumor."

In other words, he didn't find cancer. This animal, he learned, should have been treated for diabetes and heart disease. Carpenter's diagnosis had been wrong.

The aftermath was less torturous than it could have been. Had the animal lived, treatment would have been costly, and even then nothing was guaranteed. When Brum informed the owners of the mistake, he got the impression that they would have euthanized the cat anyway. "That made me feel a little better," the pathologist said, "but it's not an excuse."

The error disturbed Jim. Indirectly, he was to blame for the death of a patient. Moreover, he feared that Brum, and in turn other doctors upstairs, might lose faith in his opinions, and that he had damaged his department's reputation.

In the hubbub of daily life, most of the staff never even learned about the incident. Had they, the majority would have said that no doctor—no matter what species he treated—was perfect. It was doubtful that anyone on staff had escaped committing an error that had cost an animal its life.

They knew, too, that a pathologist's job was less cut-and-dry than it looked. The cells on any given sample could be difficult to evaluate, especially without a powerful electron microscope and the necessary technical support. The lack of expensive and short-lived diagnostic antibodies, found only at the larger research institutions, was also a handicap. Though Carpenter could send samples out, his budget for such a luxury was but a thousand dollars.

In brief, it would have required a trespass of greater magnitude, perhaps along the lines of crimes against humanity, to sully Carpenter's image of reliability.

Still, over the years, the pathologist had failed to notice identifiable diseases on a number of slides. "Sins of omission," he called them. If they came back to haunt him at all, it was usually years later, when someone was conducting a study using the old materials and happened upon the mistake.

Worse, Carpenter felt, was a misdiagnosis that caused an animal to be killed, injected with dangerous drugs, or needlessly cut open in surgery. Carpenter could recall only one such incident in which he played a part in an animal's being euthanized—Brum's patient. Though the pathologist's batting average remained high, that case made the stakes of his work exceedingly clear.

Pathology was the least glamorous section of Angell. Unlike the clinics upstairs, television crews and reporters rarely came by. Since pathology staffers spent so much time with the dead, some people saw them as ghouls. Theirs was a very precise endeavor, requiring strict adherence to protocol. ("They're majorly anal down there," is how Doug Brum put it.)

Everyone knew, however, that pathology was the final diagnostic word at Angell. And the man with the beard, Carpenter, was the final word in pathology.

It was only fitting that the department should be in the basement, for it was in many ways the foundation for all that went on upstairs. Day in and day out, the veterinary staff turned to pathology for answers. Even with the vets' radiographs and access to high-tech diagnostic equipment like ultrasound and magnetic resonance imaging, only the pathologist could provide definitive word—and as Brum's case proved, life and death hung in the balance.

To look around downstairs, one would hardly know it. At one end of the department was Carpenter's office, his desktop predictably loaded with files and paperwork. Clear down the hall was the clinical laboratory, where bodily fluids like blood, urine, bone marrow, and spinal fluid, as well as waste matter, were analyzed. It was headed by a second pathologist, Lois Roth, who had just come on board.

Carpenter spent much of his day at a light microscope—that provided viewing for as many as five people at a time—in a tight, little room that staffers regularly motored through on their way between offices. There was hardly enough space to slide back one's seat from the table. The only decoration was a bulletin board with a sign that Carp had tacked up: "You only fail when you stop trying."

Around the corner were the residents' offices. One of the pathologists in training had taped a *New Yorker* cartoon on his door. Depicted was a cat coroner reporting to some cat police officers the cause of death of yet another cat, this one laid out on the table in the background. "'Curiosity,'" read the caption.

A little farther down the corridor, technicians prepared slides for analysis. Next door in the necropsy room, residents and interns autopsied an average of one animal a day, though sometimes time and chance or a special investigation by the society's law enforcement division brought numerous dead bodies. Each corpse was examined for obvious signs of trauma or disease. Then, in workmanlike fashion, the resident or intern collected samples from the organs and various glands.

Carpenter performed his own necropsies on special cases but otherwise only came in afterward, along with his remaining trainees, for the summary of findings and evaluation. These gatherings around dissected animals were known as "demos," though some dubbed them "meat meetings."

"Vivos docent," read a wooden sign on the wall. Translated from the Latin, it said, "They teach the living."

Pathology seemed to rest only when the doors to the department were locked at the end of each day and everyone went home. Each year Carpenter and his charges analyzed thousands of biopsy slides for the veterinarians upstairs and for outside practitioners and institutions. Overall, business was up that year. Among other things, the clinical lab had added new equipment—a computer as well as a chemistry analyzer—allowing pathology to take on more work from outside practices.

"How's everything down in pathology?" one of the upstairs staffers asked Luther DeVaughn, a technician, one day when he ventured up to the first floor for a snack.

"Dead," DeVaughn said with a straight face. "Everything's dead down there."

JIM CARPENTER WAS NEWLY ENTHUSED. MIKE ARON-sohn, who headed surgery, was preparing a study on pericardial effusion in dogs. He had gone through the old pathology files—a rare resource of some eighty thousand tissue samples dating back to 1946—and pulled together every case in which the thin sac of membrane around the heart had ruptured, allowing the fluid inside to escape into the body. Then he came to Carpenter to review the cases.

It was extra work, but Carpenter did not mind. "There is no better experience than to sit down in a short time span and look at a *bunch* of something," he said excitedly, "rather than see an example of something today and another example six months from now. You can gain *a lot* by looking at a condition in a concentrated form.

"So I've gone over the cases he gave me. Now I'm going over

other cases of pericardial effusions. And when I'm through going through a-a-al-l the cases, then I'm going to go back over his group again and see if they fall into categories. I can hardly wait to go back over it again. That's gonna be the fun part, after I've got this foundation. Then I can say I looked at all the cases of pericardial effusion in dogs seen at Angell Memorial Animal Hospital since 1946. I've looked at *all* the examples, *all* the different causes!"

Carpenter's excitement was bemusing, but it was also infectious. Even if you cared not at all, and knew nothing about pericardial effusion in dogs, for example, it was impossible to remain unmoved. After all, before you was the very man who planned to view *all* the examples, *all* the causes.

Jim's nature was to ride his on-the-job experiences to the hilt. He would take a study like Aronsohn's, or any number of others, and embrace it like the assignment came from on high. Even with an error like the one with Brum's patient, Carpenter squeezed out every drop of usefulness. "I use it when teaching now," he said. "It's a learning device."

Carpenter also brought some competition, a sense of sport, to his job. Hence his pride at being the first and only to see this or accomplish that. It fed his competitive nature and kept things interesting.

He encouraged others to follow suit. His residents, for example, were told not to go home until they learned at least ten new bits of information daily. When he ran the continuing-education seminars for staff doctors and outside practitioners, he dangled bottles of non-alcoholic California rosé before them as the spoils for being first to answer his special quiz questions.

His work, however, often had its own urgency. Carpenter and his staff were integral to many investigations by the MSPCA's law enforcement division. Jim's autopsy work the previous year, in fact, had been crucial in helping the society win a sensitive case against a shelter director in Worcester who was inhumanely euthanizing animals.

From time to time, Carpenter's expertise was sought by people outside the profession. About ten years ago, attorneys for a woman who had found a mouse in her bottle of grape soda contacted him. No doubt speeding her settlement with the company, Carpenter reported in complete seriousness, "The findings of an apparently healthy, noninjured, dead mouse in a beverage bottle, the indication of fluid in the lungs, and the histological findings of hypoxia and congestion would all suggest that the mouse died as a result of the bottling process and that the mouse was alive when fluid was introduced into the bottle."

Another time, a syrup manufacturer asked him to examine another mouse corpse that a customer claimed to have found in a bottle of its product. This time Carpenter felt certain that the rodent in question got into the product long after bottling, making the company blameless. "I felt very confident," he remembered. "And what really made me mad was that after going through all this, the company decided to settle out of court. They said they didn't want the publicity."

Airlines sent him pets to necropsy that had died in their jets' baggage compartments en route to Boston's Logan International Airport. The victims tended to be short-muzzled dogs, like the pug or the bulldog. Such animals often have difficulty breathing under normal conditions; the stress of air travel, combined with hot weather and poor air circulation in the baggage section can lead to heat prostration.

Once, in 1983, an airline sent him seven dead greyhounds, all racing dogs, that had come in from Texas. "God," remembered Carpenter, "they were shipped with muzzles on. How stupid can people be? A dog's got to be able to pant, to open its mouth. They have to be given the opportunity to take deep breaths and get lots of air in a short time. People don't even use common sense."

Another time it was a Saint Bernard, also dead from hyperthermia. The dog had been transported in a huge crate but without enough ventilation. "You took the Saint Bernard out of that crate, and it was nothing but wet," Carpenter said, shaking his head. "There was an imprint for days in the bottom of that crate exactly where the body was located. That poor dog."

On any given day, anything could come through the door for autopsy. Carpenter received pets from owners who suspected malpractice by their veterinarians. A private research laboratory sent him mice that had died of a disease it never created and that was wiping out its experimental animals. Another lab sent him mice from experiments to discover whether a woman's carpet was making her ill.

One day two FBI agents strode in with what looked like the skeleton of a human foot, its toes hacked off. A dog had come out of some woods, they told him, and delivered the foot to its stunned owner. They needed to know whether this was man or beast. A better bet would have been to see someone more familiar with bones, such as a radiologist, not a veterinary pathologist. But Carpenter, who knew a thing or two about hunting, gave them his opinion, anyway: it was a bear's foot.

"When you're hunting or skinning," he said years later, "it's very difficult to get the skin off the digits. So, to make the job of skinning a bear easier, you would cut the metatarsals. The fact that someone had cut those bones about the same location told me, hell, it was a hunter, someone who had skinned deer and bear before. But, boy, that would have been a gruesome story, that someone took the time to skin a human, to cut off its toes at the same location."

Murder mysteries aside, what made Carpenter happiest was peering into his microscope and seeing diseases he had never seen before. Even better was when he encountered those that no one had seen, or at least ever reported in the literature. Over the years, he was involved in more than sixty original reports of disease, the subjects of which would be obscure to the average pet owner but which advanced veterinary medicine.

More than two decades ago, Carpenter turned to pathology in refuge from the insatiable demands of Angell's clients and their pets. Yet the attraction of pathology had always been there. As a working veterinarian, he had always felt somewhat shortchanged: rarely was there enough information. In pathology, though, he could combine everything they found upstairs and what he saw in the microscope and know what was wrong—usually, at least. Even if worse came to worst and the animal died, he always learned something.

"Who else in the hospital has this opportunity?" he demanded. "Nobody. They just see pieces. Here, we get a chance to look at the laboratory data, the X rays, the report of the radiologist, the cardiologist, the history, the physical findings, the signs the animal was showing, and then correlate all of that with the lesion."

Unlike medical pathologists, who know a lot about a single species—namely human—Carpenter and his ilk were versed in many. Angell drew plenty of samples from dogs and cats, of course, but outside veterinarians at zoological centers and research facilities also kept Carpenter and his people busy with tissues from mice, snakes, ducks, giraffes, chimpanzees, and a slew of other creatures.

Still, Carpenter admitted that these days it was harder to come across something that sat him up straight, that kept his mental engine in high gear. "I'm no longer stimulated the way I used to be," he said. "Last summer I attended a lecture at Woods Hole Oceanographic Institution on Cape Cod. It was on marine pathology. Man, did that stimulate me, because I don't get any specimens of marine animals. I could get very interested in that, or I could get very interested in commercial chickens and turkeys and pigs. The reason is that it would be new."

Over the past few decades, Carpenter had contributed substantially to his profession. He was proud of that. Yet, as his career pointed toward its close, he saw that new ground was being broken that went beyond anything he or his peers had accomplished. "If I was starting out today," he said, "I would specialize not in gross pathology, not in microscopic pathology, but molecular pathology. I'd want to look at molecules and what's responsible for making the molecule—and that's the gene.

"I could sit here today, and I could say that I know why the German shepherd and the golden retriever, with their high incidence of tumors, have defective genes. There's something wrong that predisposes them—it's the breeding. And somebody sometime in the next decade will be able to tell you exactly *why* the German shepherd is prone to developing hemangiosarcoma, say, or why the rottweiler is so susceptible to parvovirus enteritis.

"There will be many, many of these examples. And then, of course, there are people that hope to be able to change the gene from a bad one into a good one.

"That will be the final goal."

PART FOUR *Humaniacs*

Science does not embody all that men know.

—HENRY DAVID THOREAU, Journal, January 7, 1851

17
Roots

FLIERS HAD BEEN POSTED ALL OVER THE BUILDING for weeks announcing a "garden party." Still, no one from Angell save some secretaries showed up for the ceremony celebrating the 169th anniversary of MSPCA founder George Angell's birth.

After all, it was chilly for June. The wind, too, was whipping around behind the building, where the flower garden was being dedicated. The gunmetal gray skies were threatening rain. All were adequate excuses to beg off attending the informal gathering that had been organized by the society's humane services division.

The simple truth, though, was that not many people from the hospital were particularly interested.

The twenty or so MSPCA staffers in attendance, most of whom were dedicated to broader animal issues, never expected them to come in the first place. Led by Carter Luke—a rangy, bewhiskered, gentle man, adorned in a tie with a raccoon image on it—the attendees gathered around the poppies and morning glories and daylilies that Luke himself had planted and sang, with no evident embarrassment, "Happy Birthday to George" as well as an equally fervid round of the "How old are you now?" verse.

Luke sliced into the earth with a ceremonial silver shovel. Here, amidst the myriad flowers, he proceeded to plant a symbolically correct Angel Face rose. "We're not here to bury George," Luke announced to the chilled gathering. "We're here to praise him! And what's the phrase we're using?"

"WE'RE WORKING AT THE ROOTS!"

The uninitiated might have taken this as the rallying cry of an impassioned gardening club. In truth, it was among many clarion calls sounded a century ago by George Thorndike Angell, one of the nation's earliest and most prominent crusaders for a new humanity toward animals. He had started the Massachusetts Society for the Prevention of Cruelty to Animals in 1868, following similar groups in Great Britain, New York, and Philadelphia.

Angell's dream was to enlighten the masses, children in particular, about the moral wrong of maltreatment of animals. He believed he was planting the seeds for greater kindness among people and even the end of wars. As Angell put it when critics challenged his devotion to mere creatures, despite the obvious needs of mankind: "We are working at the roots."

These days, the MSPCA was behind an array of local, national, and international efforts on behalf of animals that impressed even the cynical. For example, the society supported a veterinary hospital for work animals and others in Fez, Morocco. Its affiliate the World Society for the Protection of Animals, also on the Jamaica Plain property, worked to save animals around the globe, including those endangered by war and natural disasters.

Stateside, law enforcement officers in Boston and around Massachusetts investigated thousands of cases involving animal cruelty and unsuitable living conditions. Seven shelters took in tens of thousands of unwanted pets, adopting out about eight thousand a year, but having to euthanize scores of others. Staffers from the American Humane Education Society, another affiliate, brought books and special programs about humane treatment into schools around Boston and the nation.

Other personnel pressed for legislative reform. The MSPCA

was a driving force, for instance, in passage of several amendments to the Animal Welfare Act. The organization was not flamboyant, but its tentacles touched a lot of animals—and people.

Despite the parochial sound of its name, the MSPCA had an endowment of about $54 million and stood among the world's wealthiest animal welfare organizations. A mammoth 40 percent of that endowment was restricted to Angell, the society's flagship. But truth be told, it was the Carter Lukes—not the veterinarians—who were the spiritual descendants of George Thorndike Angell. In the long run, their efforts will surely benefit more animals than the labors of the hospital workers.

For many staffers at Angell Memorial there was both an ignorance about the animal protection mission of their employer and an arrogance about their own roles. Many regarded the hospital as a separate entity, simple enough given the setup of the building on South Huntington: Angell occupied most of the basement and the first and second floors. The animal shelter, meanwhile, was at the rear of the building, and the other functions of the MSPCA were on floors three and four. (The fifth floor was for the most part closed off.)

"The MSPCA doesn't affect me at all," said surgeon Jim Boulay. "I consider myself completely separate from that. I work at Angell— I don't work for the MSPCA." A glance at his paycheck would no doubt reveal that Boulay was wrong.

Still, he was only expressing what was felt by a lot of Angell employees, who saw themselves as soldiers on the front lines in the so-called real world. "I'm here to treat the patients," snapped one Angell staffer when asked about the hospital's divergence from the humane society. "I'm not here to cut out pictures and blow up balloons."

The latter was the image a lot of hospital people had about the society's other employees. They figured those upstairs cared about animals—in a fuzzy, touchy-feely sort of way—but surmised that they worked in their bare feet all day and eschewed hamburgers for tofu. "They're all stressed out upstairs," started a common joke around Angell. "It's Whale Awareness Week." Many at Angell dismissed the humane services staffers as "humaniacs" or "granola eaters." Because the hospital's floors were polished tile and those upstairs were carpeted, a number of hospital staffers simply referred to their overhead counterparts as "the rug people."

"The MSPCA would be nothing if it wasn't for Angell Memorial," said neurologist Allen Sisson. "George Angell's ideas would be a piece of dead dust. The hospital was a fortuitous idea that kept the society alive. They may not want to admit it, but they all know it."

GEORGE ANGELL'S BEGINNINGS WERE IN SMALL-TOWN Southbridge, Massachusetts, near Worcester, where he was the only child of a Baptist pastor. When he was four, his father died, leaving George and his mother with a precarious future. His mother found sustenance work as a teacher, but much of Angell's childhood was spent living with relatives around New England.

He overcame early adversity. Between his mother's determination, the boy's own work ethic, and a number of well-placed relations, Angell graduated from Dartmouth College and became a successful Boston attorney.

At age forty-four Angell's life turned. He had long been concerned about the maltreatment of domestic animals, workhorses in particular, but in 1868 he read in the newspaper about a punishing Washington's Birthday horse race from Brighton to Worcester. The two horses were forced to pull sleds with two men each some forty miles. In the end both horses died of exhaustion—and Angell found his purpose in life.

The result was the MSPCA, which would grow into perhaps the wealthiest, most far-reaching animal welfare organization on earth. The tremendous growth came later, but Angell was the driving and unifying force that gave the society its life—and spirit. He pulled together a Brahmin board of directors and tapped every potential source of assistance.

For Angell this was a higher calling. He gave up law to devote himself to humane issues, at one point even calling himself "the advocate of the lower races." The society's emblem was an illustration of an avenging angel, sword in hand, intervening as a man goes to club a befallen horse. Beneath the nameplate on every issue of the society's propaganda organ, a periodical called *Our Dumb Animals,* were William Cowper's lines about never entering "on my list of friends . . . the man who needlessly sets foot upon a worm."

Into the early 1900s, George Angell was a renowned defender of animals, rivaled only by fellow pioneers Henry Bergh in New York and England's Richard "Humanity Dick" Martin. His organization erected drinking fountains for horses and pushed through the Massachusetts legislature stiffer laws against animal cruelty. The society's agents also prosecuted offenders.

Education, however, was Angell's main focus. He lectured and traveled widely. He helped establish humane organizations around the country. He joined in forming the American Bands of Mercy, a national youth organization that encouraged kindness toward animals and humans. He founded the American Humane Education Society (AHES) to bring the same message into the schools and churches.

Furthermore, for what he saw as a larger good, Angell simply pirated *Black Beauty.* Written by Anna Sewell, the book had been published in England to some success. Angell regarded it as his movement's answer to *Uncle Tom's Cabin.* Since Sewell had died and only her publisher seemed likely to gain, Angell's AHES published it without authorization. Hundreds of thousands of copies were distributed free or sold inexpensively, in American and foreign editions, to a great extent making *Black Beauty* a classic and, of course, advancing Angell's cause.

This was an age of do-good societies and reformers, but Angell still seemed outlandish, particularly early on. Once when he went to speak, the audience erupted in laughter when his topic—cruelty to animals—was announced. Abolitionist William Lloyd Garrison, a fanatic for another cause, vowed in the pages of his *Liberator,* "I WILL BE HEARD." So it was for Angell, only the MSPCA's vehicle was *Our Dumb Animals* (the title, referring, of course, to an inability to talk). "We speak for those who cannot speak for themselves" was the paper's righteous motto.

"We have a three-fold work before us," Angell wrote. "First, to protect dumb animals; second, to convert human brutes into merciful men; third, to educate the children—to teach them that God created and cares for every living thing; that cruelty to the defenseless is not only mean and cowardly, but in direct conflict with the principles of Christianity, and leading on to all that is bad and wicked in the state."

With his silvery hair and beard, Angell personified the MSPCA. As the years passed, *Our Dumb Animals* increasingly reflected Angell's feelings on a variety of issues, such as his Victorian-era angst about the possibility of premature burial. Angell also took aim at larger human issues, such as adulterated foods, the dangers of lead, and the tragedy of war. Yet, he never strayed from animal concerns for very long.

He delighted in one editor's comparing him to "an old clock which once wound up would never stop striking." In his writing, Angell belittled the mighty and those he regarded as warmongers and enemies to animals, though it is doubtful that his targets much cared. He lambasted Benjamin Harrison and Theodore Roosevelt for, among other things, participating in blood sports. In 1908 he editorialized against William H. Taft for president: "*If our clients,* the horses, could vote," he began, "we don't believe they would vote for a man said to weigh *over three hundred pounds* who rides horseback."

Henry Bergh, famous for his work in New York as president of the American Society for the Prevention of Cruelty to Animals, wrote to Angell, "I have seen you spoken of by the Press here, as 'an Angell of mercy.' You are earning the title."

As fiery as Angell appeared, he was sensitive as well. When his pet canary, which flew free in Angell's apartment and even came when called, was killed by a cat, the MSPCA's leader was devastated. He wrote that to have lost a thousand dollars' worth of possessions would have been comparatively inconsequential. "What there is beyond the dark river we know not," Angell wrote, "but we humbly hope this little bird life, which has brought so much happiness into our home during the past five years, may not have gone out forever."

When Angell himself crossed that river, he was eighty-six years old. Thirty-eight workhorses, black rosettes attached to their bridles, trailed his hearse through the streets of Boston before the burial at Mount Auburn Cemetery in Cambridge. Newspapers around the nation, which had received *Our Dumb Animals* for years, eulogized him. The *Malden* (Massachusetts) *Mail* wrote: "All the dumb animals would mourn if they knew of the death of the president of the Society for the Prevention of Cruelty to Animals, Angell in name, angel in nature."

FRANCIS H. ROWLEY MADE NO PRETENSIONS OF being the second coming of George Angell when he succeeded the MSPCA's founder in 1910. Instead, the former Baptist minister brought new energy and furthered the cause of the humane movement by evoking the name of Angell, "the apostle of humanity to animals," at every turn.

Rowley was a short, kindly gentleman, a scholar. His father was a physician, and Rowley himself held a doctor of divinity degree, ingredients that gave him a unique perspective. With his bald pate, round gold-rimmed spectacles, and full white mustache, he was the picture of grandfatherly benevolence.

During the four decades that Rowley held the job, he would stamp his approval on numerous projects bearing Angell's name, from a towering memorial and watering fountain for horses in Boston's Post Office Square, to a school, to a liberty ship. Nothing, however, that Rowley achieved matched in foresight his decision shortly after he became president to press for the construction of Angell Memorial Animal Hospital.

At his death, George Angell's own dreams were less elaborate. He simply wished that his two organizations, the MSPCA and the American Humane Education Society, would someday be housed in the same structure, "The Humane Building." Shortly after he died, the board of directors sought to raise funds for that purpose. By the time of Rowley's ascension, however, the humane movement had grown up. Some said Angell's MSPCA, now financially well off, had grown "quiescent." Medical care for animals, meanwhile, was coming into its own, and Boston lagged behind. Rowley noted that a number of animal hospitals were well established abroad. Perhaps more important, the late Bergh's ASPCA had opened a busy animal hospital and shelter in New York, as had the New York Women's League for Animals.

"This is the latest phase of humane work," Rowley wrote of veterinary medicine. "It is one more step forward. Once it was just to protect the animal from his tormentors. Now, to care for him when sick or injured, if his value to his owner warrants it, is demanded by a deepening sense of what humanity and kindness mean."

And so it was built, a memorial structure to Angell that housed the animal hospital as well as the parent organizations. By the time it was over, construction would strap the MSPCA to the tune of $250,000. Angell Memorial Animal Hospital opened in the winter of 1915 to great acclaim. "It is a rare distinction that Boston now has— the possession of the best and largest animal hospital in the world," wrote *The Boston Post*. It was constructed of brick and limestone and fronted with four granite columns topped with Ionic capitals. Its address was 180 Longwood Avenue, in the heart of the city's burgeoning medical district, which included Harvard Medical School and the Peter Bent Brigham Hospital.

When first opened, the hospital was primarily to be for horses, then so integral to daily life. There was a special operating room, electric and horse-drawn ambulances, and stalls for recovering equines, yet the cat and dog wards also were bustling. Veterinary medicine was coming into its own in the United States, particularly for small animals. The advent of the automobile signaled the gradual disappearance of the horse from everyday life. Veterinarians, who had long scorned dogs and cats, now turned to them for their livelihood.

At Boston's Angell Memorial, they did not have to look far. Pet owners, it seemed, had been waiting for such a place. From the beginning, the hospital overflowed with patients—a million would come by 1948. Expansion was constant, be it a new isolation ward or the pathology department.

Angell's veterinarians, meanwhile, capitalized on the shift toward small animals with breakthroughs in medical procedures, pinpointing new diseases, and programs. Canine hip dysplasia, for example, was diagnosed with X rays for the first time at Angell. This was among the first places to practice aseptic surgery on small animals. The Schroeder-Thomas splint, developed at Angell, was for years a mainstay for repairing fractures. Rowley had sensed that great changes were in the offing for veterinary medicine; people were ready to go to some length to obtain medical care for their creatures.

At the same time, though, Rowley was a true believer in humane education. Like George Angell, he started organizations, such as the Jack London Club, that focused on the abuse of animals in entertainment, such as circuses. He was one of the forces behind the national Be Kind to Animals Week. Toward the end of Rowley's life, Oglethorpe University in Georgia opened a school of humanities in his name.

Angell Memorial Animal Hospital, however, quickly overshadowed those broader humane activities. After all, it directly touched people and their pets. It made for good newspaper and magazine stories. It attracted celebrities, of various species. The hospital became a tremendous source of large gifts and bequeathals, a direct link to donors that other humane organizations forever lacked.

In some ways Angell Memorial was too popular. Lines of waiting clients and their pets sometimes stretched into the street. No one was turned away for an inability to pay; the MSPCA made up the difference. By the sixties the waiting room was often so crowded that only the sickest animals were treated. People literally begged doctors to see their pets. An arrogance developed, with some staffers regarding the clients and their pets almost as enemies.

For years the Longwood Avenue building was impractical, with sick animals being transported up and down staircases and a creaky elevator. Parking was impossible. And the clients and staffers who found parking places were often rewarded by having their cars stolen.

The building was deteriorating as well. "The wards were old, and the cages were rickety, and there were cockroaches at night," said former intern Richard Anderson. "I mean lots of them. It had a certain flavor to it."

Tight conditions brought a bunker comradery but also led to surreal situations. Once one doctor was in an examination room trying to steer a client toward euthanizing his dog, while in the next room two interns were joking about their favorite methods of accomplishing the very same thing. Said one, in the tones of a Southern evangelist, "I tell them that 'The *Lo-o-ord* wants your dog by His side!'" He began repeating the phrase, louder and louder, until through the thin walls, the desolate client heard shouting that for all he knew came from on high: "The *Lo-o-ord* wants your dog by His side! The *Lo-o-ord* wants your dog by His side!"

By the seventies change was inevitable. The MSPCA paid the Archdiocese of Boston two million dollars for a onetime seminary in Jamaica Plain, then spent another four and a half million dollars on renovations. The old building was sold to Harvard Medical School. The new hospital and, upstairs, the society's offices opened for business in 1976.

Not all was well, however. Angell was expensive, and it lost money—hundreds of thousands of dollars each year—for the non-profit MSPCA, largely because so much of its care was charitable.

Moreover, veterinary medicine never became the integral part of the humane movement that Rowley predicted. Nationally, the two matured separately, and Angell, a full-service animal hospital operated by a humane organization, remained unique.

Veterinary medicine, after all, was rooted in the sciences, with vivisection (animal experimentation) a standard in training. While veterinarians took care of people's pets, they were also key players in the meat industry, horse and dog racing, and research.

The humane movement, on the other hand, was philosophically based. Its concerns—from animals as food to bullfights to shelters—tended to be sweeping ethical matters that revolved around the dignity of animals. The closest link humane societies usually had to veterinary medicine was in providing free vaccinations or low-cost spaying and neutering.

What kept the MSPCA together was the decision early on to not take a wholesale stand against vivisection. It was felt that this was a battle that would only alienate people and stir dissension within the organization. Instead, the MSPCA called for moderation in using animals for research. Some saw it as weak-hearted, but the strategy paid off.

By the late seventies and eighties, however, the differences within the organization became sharper, as animal rights gained momentum nationwide. The MSPCA remained middle-of-the-road or conservative, avoiding the protests and wild publicity stunts that became common in the animal movement.

Clearly, though, Angell and its veterinarians were increasingly being called to task by their humane-services brethren. Conflicts arose, for example, over the ethics of using shelter animals as blood donors for the hospital. Disputes came up over the use of euthanized animals' corpses to practice surgical techniques or for studies on such organs as the thyroid. Veterinarians were ordered to give up consulting for organizations involved in animal research. Declawing cats, regarded by humane workers as merely a convenience to owners, was banned at Angell and the newer MSPCA hospitals in Springfield and Nantucket.

Arguments flared over fund allocations. Sometimes infighting even erupted over the menus—vegetarian fare or meat—at society-wide workshops and banquets. Hard feelings were common. At one point, there was even talk of unloading Angell by selling it to the fledging veterinary school at Tufts—for a dollar.

Tension mounted within Angell, as well. Salaries were too low. One longtime staff veterinarian took legal action, arguing that she was underpaid because of her gender, which spun out into her being fired and a nasty lawsuit that remained unresolved for years. What's more, many felt that Angell Memorial, once a leader in its field, had fallen too far behind the now pace-setting veterinary schools.

Outside critics were also vocal. To some the MSPCA was a lumbering giant that hoarded its wealth and was always a step or two behind other animal activists. A common complaint was that Angell failed to provide enough financial assistance, though in truth few animal hospitals anywhere provided so much. Meanwhile, other humane organizations argued that the society was lax in reacting to dog and cat overpopulation concerns.

Critics also found it hard to believe that the society had financial woes. However, the society's endowment, which by mid-1996 was at $54 million, had been dipped into so often that it lagged behind the inflation rate. The nonprofit's financial people blanched when they saw that in real terms the MSPCA was eating away its future.

The new building, for instance, may have relieved many of the day-to-day stresses on Angell Memorial, but it was also the first of several big-ticket costs to reverberate through the MSPCA's coffers for years. Around the time of the move, veterinary medicine and technology slowly improved, and costs skyrocketed. Between the limitations on what an animal hospital could expect a pet owner to pay and the long-standing policy to provide free care to those in need, Angell was spending nearly half of the MSPCA's annual budget and losing more than a million dollars a year.

The MSPCA was far from poor, but its widespread activities spread allocations thin. More than anything, its fiscal house needed better controls, especially to keep the endowment, which was smaller than those of many colleges, healthy. Former Angell chief of staff Gus Thornton, a man of tremendous girth, was elevated to the society's presidency in 1989. A fixture around the hospital since his internship in 1957, Thornton's mission now was to unify the society and to stop the endowment from bleeding.

Some on the humane issues side of the organization fretted at the thought of a veterinarian at the helm. But not long after taking the job, Thornton opened a lot of eyes by publicly speaking out for curbs on animal research, flying in the face of many of his longtime friends and colleagues. As for his own organization, Thornton now demanded budget tightening across the board, Angell included.

Thornton would draw criticism for his salary, which hovered around $175,000, with a hefty life insurance policy, and use of a company car. Indeed, the entire matter of executive salaries was a touchy one for the MSPCA—and many other non-profits. Potential donors who envisioned their hard-earned dollars going to the care of doe-eyed dogs and cats stood to be turned off when they learned what the top dog, Thornton, took home every year.

In his defense, Thornton was an institution around the MSPCA. And for better or worse, his pay was in line with the top executives of similar nonprofits. Yet, the critics countered, *no one* who works for a charity should expect to grow rich.

That said, Thornton was an important player for the MSPCA. He understood the society's internal divisions and made an effort to bring the sides together. He wanted the humane aspects to become stronger and, where possible, more self-sustaining. He saw to it, too, that new veterinarians and interns at least learned about the larger aspects of the society, and he encouraged them to get involved.

Change was slowly occurring. A few of the younger staff doctors and interns, Lynne Morris among them, were active allies of the humane cause, helping with special programs or lending their skills to the shelter. But those veterinarians were in the minority. Most people at Angell held fast to their doubts about the "humaniacs" upstairs. Singing songs and dedicating gardens to a long-dead founder was fine, they decided, so long as attendance was optional. In the end, that suited those on the third and fourth floors as well. To each his own, after all.

Still, even the humane workers became a little sheepish when they recalled the year they decided to go en masse, at lunch, to honor Angell's birthday at his gravesite. A cemetery official came by to explain that picnicking on the grounds was prohibited, but his instructions were somehow misunderstood. By the second time, the man simply had enough of these famished animal lovers and felt it necessary to take matters into his own hands.

To this day there are still some MSPCA staffers who grow red-faced when they recall the scene, for that was the fateful day when the philosophical sons and daughters of George Angell were expelled from Mount Auburn Cemetery.

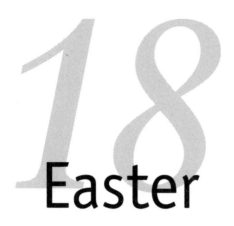

Easter

BY ITS VERY NATURE, THE OVERNIGHT SHIFT WAS depressing. Adding to it, the night before Easter had settled in drizzly and chilly. Lynne Morris couldn't help but wish to be a little happier. It was one of those days, and one of those nights, when fate handed the intern a series of lost causes, animals so far gone that she could do little more than make their final hours a bit more comfortable, then turn out the lights and wrap up the paperwork.

That afternoon she lost a rabbit—a "bunny" in Morris's vernacular—that had come in half dead, probably a reaction to chemicals used by a groomer. The owner had wanted the animal looking its best for a storefront display on Easter morning. When she got it home, though, the rabbit began having seizures and could not walk. By the time the owner arrived at Angell, it was already too late. Lynne checked the rabbit into intensive care, but it was dead by Saturday afternoon.

Anyone who has worked around shelters and animal hospitals knows about Easter. Traditionally, that is when a lot of well-meaning parents give their children live rabbits and, sometimes, chicks to celebrate the holiday. Then as early as a day or two later, when the children become bored with the pets, those same parents come by to surrender the animals—that is, if the creatures had not met a worse fate of mistreatment or inadequate care or being set loose in the neighborhood.

Morris knew a bit more than most young veterinarians about shelters. In veterinary school she spent her externships at Boston's Animal Rescue League and the Michigan Humane Society, where they needed help with spays and neuters and shots. In Michigan, in fact, she adopted one of her dogs, Graham, a German shepherd mix that had to have one of his legs amputated after suffering a gunshot wound. At Angell Morris helped out in the shelter when she could. She was painfully aware of the thousands of unwanted animals—most of them perfectly healthy—that were euthanized, piled into barrels, and incinerated.

For Morris, Saturday night and Sunday morning continued the cavalcade of forsaken sick and injured animals: a seizing golden retriever; a cage of baby hamsters, all dead or dying; a three-legged stray mongrel, soaking wet, with a back so broken after being struck by a car that when Morris ran her fingers over its spine, she felt a two-inch dropoff at the break.

At midnight Lynne had ushered a young Hispanic couple and their little girl, just five or six years old, into an exam room. They had traveled from the distant northern suburbs in hopes of saving their daughter's rabbit, Gucci, which the mother held wrapped in a baby blanket in her arms.

Morris examined the rabbit, an albino. She opened its mouth and pressed a finger against its gums. A healthy animal's gums would be pink and change from pink to white to pink again at the pressure of an examining touch. Gucci's were mostly white. Its temperature, meanwhile, was down. The animal was emaciated and dehydrated, probably from the diarrhea it had been enduring for more than a week. "Her condition is not very good right now," Lynne explained to the family. "If she makes it through the night, maybe . . ."

By a quarter to three Easter morning, the night people and their pets seemed to have finally tapped themselves out. The hour had grown tranquil as the hospital somnolently buzzed and hummed.

For Lynne Morris, it was coming-down time. She found herself sitting on a hard, orange plastic chair in F ward, the small room that houses Angell's exotics, in this case, a rabbit named Gucci. Lynne was in her hospital whites, and on her lap was the dying rabbit, which antibiotics, hot water bottles to help raise its temperature, and all else were too late to help.

"Her pretty pink eyes are blue now," Morris said. "That's not good. She's not getting any oxygen." Melancholy, she pressed a finger against the animal's gums: white. She pressed her stethoscope against its underside and heard the faintest of heartbeats.

A minute later there was none. "I'm batting a thousand with my bunnies today," was all Morris said.

She rose and stepped into the hall. Around the corner was a gurney where dead animals were tagged and left to be gathered and disposed of by an attendant. She set Gucci down, took some files, and made her way across the empty waiting room, up a darkened hallway, and into the front office to make a telephone call. "Hello," she said to an answering machine, "this is Dr. Morris. I'm afraid we have some bad news . . ."

When she hung up, hospital supervisor Bob Bassett told her how the little girl had been weeping and carrying on about the animal when the family arrived. "I only billed them eighty-five dollars to check it in overnight," he said. "I didn't have the heart to ask for what we usually want." He shook his head. "It's not going to be a happy Easter for that little girl."

"Well," said Morris, "they can come to the shelter Tuesday and get all the bunnies they want."

19

Hunter

WITH THE ARRIVAL OF PLEASANT WEATHER, JIM
Carpenter allowed himself the luxury of occasionally letting his mind
drift away from his microscope. From the head-high windows in the
necropsy room, he could see the cloudless skies and the lawn coming
in thick and lush. After work most nights he would sit on a picnic
table behind his home in suburban Dedham, swallow a couple shots
of whiskey, rub down his insistent cat Otis, who invariably joined
him, and contemplate the domain that was his yard, his flower garden,
and, as the year wore on, his tomato plants.

The new season also awakened a spirit in him that few within
the hospital or MSPCA could ever understand. Carpenter, after all,
was an outdoorsman, a not-so-endearing appellation in an organization long opposed to the destruction of animals for sport. He had
been raised in rural Wisconsin and was passionate about being out on
a small boat with his children (he had six, now all grown), or his siblings, fishing for pickerel or bass; stepping through the woods, shotgun in hand, hunting deer; or marking time in a blind for his chance
to bag a duck.

Though others in the organization—including president Gus Thornton—were avid fishermen, most frowned upon hunters. Some people made sarcastic remarks behind the pathologist's back, but rarely did anyone complain about his pastimes to his face. "I'm a hunter," Carpenter stamped when asked about it. "They don't *dare* tell me I can't hunt. I'd tell them what to do in a minute."

These days Carpenter's thoughts often drifted to the Charles River, which snaked through Boston's western suburbs. Some days he brought to Angell a silver fishing bucket filled with water and minnows, so that he could head straight out after work without even having to stop at a bait store. In fact, he kept the shiners in the giant cooling unit where dead animals awaited autopsy; the cold helped keep the bait viable.

Because Carpenter seldom socialized and his basement office was off the beaten trail, many at Angell could go weeks without seeing him. Following a spring rain, though, fellow employees occasionally spied Jim wandering slowly around the parking lot and the lawn, head stooped, steadfastly searching for something. "The only interaction I've ever had with this guy was in the parking lot, because we both arrive around the same time," said ICU nurse Joan Fontaine. "He waves to me, I wave to him. Every time he sees me, he gives me this big wave and a smile. I don't even know his first name.

"One time he was out there looking in the grass, and I figured, 'Well, he probably dropped his keys.' So I go to help him. I'm out there looking and looking; we're both looking. Finally, I said, 'Well, where'd you drop 'em?' And he says, 'Drop what?' I said, 'Your keys.' He said, 'I didn't lose my keys.' I said, 'Well, then what are you lookin' for?' He goes, 'Night crawlers; I'm going fishin'.'"

That was how most people at the hospital knew Carpenter: through brief sightings and bits and pieces of conversation. Even Paul Gambardella and other longtime staffers, who had relied on Jim's expertise for years, rarely learned much that was personal. He reported every morning to work, and work he did—relentlessly, like a galley slave.

As the years passed, he perhaps had become too isolated.

Gambardella felt that pathology had become too much of its own island, not interacting as much as he would like with the rest of the staff. Carpenter, he said, daunted many of the younger doctors, which only added to the problem. "Right now, whether he knows it or not, Jim is very intimidating to the staff," Paul said. "For the Gambardellas and the old-timers, there's no problem, but the new people are scared to death of that man."

It was general knowledge that Carp was an emotional, opinionated individual, but most people only knew about his impassioned outbursts at staff meetings and the like. (Once he even stunned onlookers by roaring in a complaint about some failing of Favorite Son Doug Brum.)

On Monday afternoons, which he set aside to be interviewed for this book, another Jim Carpenter emerged. This one, too, was powered by strong emotions. Certain subjects, like the hospital's incentive plan and Angell's need for strong leadership, could have him growling almost instantly. Other topics—his upbringing, his early years at the hospital, his accomplishments—set him off on jags of nostalgia and pride.

What seemed to make him happiest—outside of contemplating the intricacies of animal diseases—was recollecting his tromps through the wooded mountains of New Hampshire, stalking deer. Since the late sixties, it was one of the select pleasures Carpenter afforded himself. Every fall he and Vern Caron, who worked in the MSPCA's purchasing department and who died of cancer several years ago, spent about five days hunting, often with some outside friends. Over the years Carpenter bagged four deer, each with a single blast. He still betrayed a hunter's natural ebullience when recounting his biggest kill, a weighty eleven-point buck. Like most hunters, Carpenter spoke often of the natural splendors he saw on those expeditions, de-emphasizing the killing. He liked to recall, for instance, the panoramic view from the upper reaches of Mount Orn: Carpenter and his friends could drink in the glory of Mount Washington to the north; to the east, Franconia Notch; the Connecticut River, meanwhile, rolled on to the west, drawing the boundary between New

Hampshire and Vermont. Sometimes when the sky was clear, a pair of binoculars brought into focus a distant railroad line, often with a train chugging along. "And last year, a couple of jet planes, fighters, were playing tag down through the valley," Carpenter remembered. "Honestly, I was higher than the jets. That was beautiful."

Hunting also provided a unique comradery. Often on those trips, Caron and Carp would separate to better cover the territory. On their own, each would instinctively be drawn to some scenic lookout point or another. Sensing that the other would find his way there, too, the first arrival would leave a teasing note, much like a schoolkid. It was a small matter—silliness, even—but it was the stuff that cements friendships and that now triggered a wave of memories and emotions for Carpenter.

One afternoon, as he talked about those notes and the rustic beauty he enjoyed so much, Jim Carpenter laughed easily. Quickly, though, he grew solemn and embarrassedly looked away. He was crying. An awkward silence filled his office. "It must be the medication for my back," he said lamely.

After a minute he gave me a hard stare. "I think you should know," he said, "that you can't always know the reasons that a person responds emotionally to something." He waved his hand: next question.

HOME—THE HOME OF JIM CARPENTER'S HEART—WAS Palmyra, Wisconsin, a rural village of fewer than a thousand people, located forty miles outside of Milwaukee. When Jim was growing up, his family lived on three different farms there, all within a mile and a half of one another. His father, Otto, was a sharecropping dairy farmer, a blacksmith, and later a machinist—doing whatever it took to pull his wife (whose struggles with mental illness required special care), and brood of kids through the Depression and other lean years that followed. Otto Carpenter had six children—four boys and two girls—with Jim being the second oldest. All of them inherited an indefatigable work ethic from the old man.

When the family's finances were bleakest, Otto would drive

into town under the cover of night and toss pebbles at the window of the fellow who owned the general store, awakening him to ask for food on credit. The kids, too, would chip in to help. Carp himself plucked turkeys for the neighbors at a quarter apiece and raised cucumbers, selling them along the roadside.

That was in addition to the regular farm duties expected of all the children. "During the summer we used to get up in the morning and get the cows to pasture, feed the cows, help carry milk, cool the milk down quickly, stir it by hand in the milk tank," Carpenter recalled. "When we weren't going to school, we'd do that, but when we were going to school, Dad would let us sleep. School came first to Dad. But then after school he'd get mad at me because I'd go right to work on the farm without changing my clothes. I just loved to work."

Hunting and fishing were as natural as the seasons in the world of Jim Carpenter's youth. In the summer his father would sometimes declare it too hot to labor and dispatch his children to the nearest creek to fish. When the kids were old enough to cover for him, the old man would set aside a day or two for hunting. Sometimes he would take the boys along. "When I was too young to carry a gun, which in my dad's opinion was less than twelve, I used to be a dog," Carpenter said. "You know what I mean? My dad and I would walk along, and I would try to scare up birds for him and then bring back pheasants."

Jim had his own dog, too: a twenty-five-pound, low-riding black mongrel named Tiny that had a mania for yanking bedsheets off of sleeping children and slogging through swamps to retrieve dead game birds. When he came of age, Carpenter and Tiny would take to the woods with his first gun, a twelve-gauge, J.C. Higgins, Sears Roebuck special, that Carpenter bought with his cucumber money.

By adulthood all of the Carpenter siblings had done well for themselves and remained friends, even though physical distance kept them apart. Brother Doug was a policeman, for example, and brother Don a highly acclaimed teacher and principal. Each of those brothers, Jim proudly reported, had shaken hands with a U.S. president—Doug, when George Bush's last campaign came to town, and

Don, when he and other outstanding educators were honored by Ronald Reagan. "I feel kind of left out of it," the pathologist said with a laugh.

Even though he never pressed presidential flesh, Jim maintained high regard within the family, being the first to go to college, at the University of Wisconsin, and then venturing even farther to attend veterinary school in Iowa. His brother Doug, in grammar school when Jim went off to learn veterinary medicine, said Jim would come home for vacations with blisters on his fingers from writing so much in his studies. "I always remember that about him," said Doug. "When he came home from school, all he did was work, read, and study."

Years later Jim joined Doug in the Canadian wilderness on a moose-hunting expedition. At one point the brothers made their way to a secluded lake that was hours from the nearest home. Doug later recalled floating in their little boat, both men thoroughly enjoying the beauty and tranquillity all around: "We were drifting along, and Jim said to me, 'Do you know that I work with people who wouldn't even believe a place like this exists? It would scare them.' You see, people from the city don't understand what it can be like to be in a place where if you sit quietly, you hear nothing, absolutely nothing."

Jim Carpenter had come from simple beginnings, yet he was among the most complex individuals at big-city Angell Memorial. The electrical charges within his brain, it often seemed, fired more rapidly than in the average human. His brilliance as a scientist, his quick intellect, and his potential for sudden and explosive mood changes made him difficult to gauge. At management meetings, for instance, no one could predict Carpenter's reaction to a proposed policy or change. Consistently, though, he would ask the most penetrating questions, which oftentimes no one else had even considered.

But it was Carpenter's more simple ways that often set him apart. In a world gone mad, no place was stranger, he often thought, than his own place of employment. Having come from a farming and scientific background, Carpenter was often miffed by some of the restrictions imposed on Angell by the MSPCA. Many of the veterinarians disagreed with the society's ban on declawing cats and curtailed use of shelter animals as blood donors, but in the end they bowed to the society's humane reasoning. Carpenter, though, was forever incredulous as to how such ethereal questions about an animal's dignity, for instance, could get in the way of *saving* others.

Carpenter simply refused to deal with what seemed like nonsense. "Now *this* is an example of the stupidity of some people who work for humane organizations, a great example of stupidity," he said one day as he marched into a storeroom and returned with an aluminum crate the size of a toaster. On its side, it read, "KETCH-ALL Automatic Mouse Trap, No Bait Needed."

"There was a hell of a mouse problem down here in pathology," he went on. "They were getting into supplies and chewing boxes. So, I ordered rodent control. And with all seriousness, they sent down some of these traps. And *I* said, 'Let's get serious! Let's use what everybody else with common sense would use, and that's called rodent poison!' Well, they finally did. But they didn't even want to poison a mouse."

He looked at the trap as if it were an ugly bug. "I didn't even know how this thing works. I just took one look at it and blew my top."

Another time, a fellow veterinarian asked him to drop by her house out in the country to rid her barn of some squirrels that had become a nuisance. As expected, Carpenter took care of the problem with his rifle. Unbeknownst to Jim, however, word got back to a leader of the MSPCA's sister organization the World Society for the Protection of Animals (WSPA). After work one day, as Carpenter was heading across the parking lot, he thought he heard someone shouting. When he looked, he saw clients and their pets, as usual, coming and going. But there also, to his bewilderment, was WSPA's John Walsh, a renowned animal advocate, yelling at him, "Killer! Killer! Killer!"

Confused and having an appointment, Carpenter shook his head, pulled out of the parking lot, and drove off. Soon afterward, he learned that his squirrel extermination project had been the reason for the attack. "Oh, was I mad," Carpenter said. "I promised myself that the next time I saw John Walsh, I'd let him have it, I'd let him know how I felt.

"Well, the next time happened to be in a department store in Dedham. He was with his wife, but I keep a promise to myself. I walked up to him, and I said, 'John, the next time you call me a killer, I'm gonna hit you right in your damn mouth!' Well, you should have seen his wife. But I was pissed."

Everyone knew that Jim Carpenter was a man of conviction in his everyday relationships and his work habits. And for all his enthusiasm about tissues, cells, tumors, and all else that blossomed in the eyepiece of his microscope, a large part of Carpenter's heart still longed to return to a simpler place. "I would like to do something different before I die," he admitted. "I really would. I don't look forward to doing this and then finding myself dead. I would like to work, even if it was for minimum wage, on a farm. I would really like to get back to nature. The only way I can do it now, it seems, is with a gun or a fishing rod. I enjoy both of them, but I still think . . .

"Well, like today: I was eating peas for lunch. People come by and laugh at me. Hell, on the farm we used to have one thing for a meal: string beans, sweet corn, field corn. We used to be happy eating mainly one thing for a meal. So for me to open a can of peas and eat the whole can for lunch doesn't bother me." Then he grinned. "But it makes everyone else sick."

ONE WEEK AFTER OUR DISCUSSION OF HUNTING AND Carpenter's tears, we met again for an hour or two. When there were no more questions and outside the sun had dropped to just above the horizon, Jim got up to return to his labors. But first he had something for me.

"Remember last time we talked, when I told you about how a person reacts emotionally? Remember I told you about the time Vern and I left notes in the woods? And I told you, you never know the reasons why a person reacts a certain way?"

I nodded.

He handed me a white piece of paper, folded once. "Don't open it now," he said. Our meeting over, he left the room.

When I finally unfolded the paper, I found it to be a photocopy of an obituary from a Wisconsin newspaper. "Services Today for Phoenix Principal," read the headline. Several years old, the piece was about Jim's brother Don, an esteemed middle school principal in Wisconsin.

Fifty-year-old Don Carpenter, the article said, had been killed in a deer-hunting accident. He was perched in a tree when the branch apparently broke, sending both Don and his weapon crashing to the earth. The gun somehow discharged, shooting Jim's brother just below the heart.

"At 6:58 a.m., on Sunday, Carpenter was spotted by the pilot of an Air National Guard helicopter in the Pine Island public hunting grounds," read the article. "He was found beneath a tree, with his Marlin lever-action rifle next to his body. Carpenter was pronounced dead at the scene."

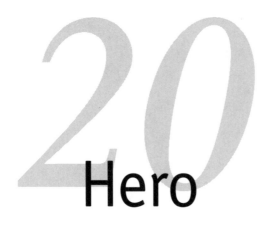

Hero

THE CALL FROM THOMAS PERKINS CAME IN TO THE MSPCA's Boston shelter one day in mid-June. Over the past six months or so, shelter staffer Amy Knapp had developed a fondness for the elderly man in Dorchester. As was the case today, Knapp had been summoned periodically to Perkin's tough, inner-city neighborhood to gather up his German shepherd, now a geriatric himself, and ferry him to Angell.

Five years earlier King had been the toast of the humane society. At an awards banquet at a posh hotel in downtown Boston, he was honored as the MSPCA's hero dog of the year. What King had done to deserve such praise was to hurl himself, fangs first, into an armed miscreant who tried to bull his way into Perkins's home and rob him. The dog took four bullets defending his master and joined Perkins in sending the terrified hoodlum crashing through a second-floor window in flight.

Nursed back to health at Angell Memorial, King received the MSPCA's royal treatment. All the local television stations reported on King, and newspapers around the country picked up the story of

Boston's canine hero. Get-well cards and letters, many with donations for King's medical bill, poured in. Besides the accolades, the MSPCA promised King free medical treatment for the rest of his days.

Now in his later years—King was most likely twelve to fifteen years old—he needed that care more and more. The previous autumn a mass was discovered in his spleen, which surprisingly turned out not to be cancer but a raging infection. In May he came in for severe pneumonia. Through it all, it was increasingly clear that King's hind legs could hardly carry him anymore.

It was afternoon when Knapp wheeled the white van—"MSPCA, On the Move for Animals" written across the side in green letters—onto Intervale Street and in front of the triple-decker where Perkins lived. Outside was the old man, with his dog stretched out on the ground, refusing to rise.

King was a sizable dog. The first thing most people noticed was that his skull was as large as a man's. He weighed one hundred pounds, with a big black muzzle, alert pointy ears, and eyes that some thought betrayed an almost human intelligence.

Knapp, who was in her early thirties, went over and chatted with the old man and sized up King's situation. As often happens with ailing dogs, the excitement of a stranger's presence overrode his pain and King arose, albeit gingerly. Knapp rigged a stretcher to serve as a ramp to the back of the van. With Perkins's help, she guided the dog inside.

Perkins, usually ebullient, was somber. Earlier, King had mis-stepped and tumbled down the stairs from his second-floor apartment. A home-remedy concoction from back in Perkins's native Georgia did the dog no good. And when the old man spoke to his children, all adults now, he glumly admitted that King was struggling. Still, merely to suggest that King might soon die stirred Perkins to anger, to the point that his kids hesitated to mention it more than once. "Don't be saying that word!" he shouted. "King ain't gonna die!"

Yet Knapp saw something in his expression that late spring day that suggested he knew otherwise. "I think in the back of his mind, he knew that the dog wasn't going to be coming back," she said. "I don't think he actually wanted to know that it was time, because of what the dog had done for him, but from the look on his face, I think he knew in his heart."

Knapp slammed the doors shut and climbed in the van. Someone from the hospital would be in touch, she told Perkins before saying her farewells, then pulling out.

BALD AND SLIGHTLY BENT WITH AGE, THOMAS PERKINS was a true character. He was a cross—both in appearance and in spirit—between the late comedian Redd Foxx and boxer George Foreman. He would turn eighty-three that year, and though slowed by time and a life of physical labor, he remained quick with the verbal comebacks, social commentary, and colorful stories.

Over his life, Perkins farmed, drove a truck, and labored at both a factory and a shipyard, among other jobs, before retiring in the late 1970s. "I done everything," he said. "You can't name the work I didn't do."

Now Perkins lived alone in Boston's crime-soaked Dorchester neighborhood, hard by another embattled section, Roxbury. He had a big family—eleven children, twenty-two grandchildren, and thirty-two great-grandchildren. His wife and most of his friends and siblings were dead, though. He had arthritis and a heart condition. The door to his apartment had four heavy-duty locks and a chain that stretched across it. At night he could hear the gangs trading gunfire and the wail of sirens. The *Boston Globe,* in fact, would one day run a page-one story about Intervale Street and its environs, calling it "a neighborhood held hostage." That was hardly news to Perkins. "They shoot folk out there and kill 'em like rabbits," he told me. "They don't care. And the police don't do nothin'."

The street thugs referred to Perkins as "Uncle Tom," an insulting play on his name. He ignored them, though, and went on his way. "The drug dealers, they don't mess with me," he said. "I got no trouble with nobody, no hollering at me, no nothin'. They call me Uncle Tom, and that's it."

Owning his own place, he was better off than many people his age. He collected Social Security and rent from the apartment downstairs. His children, however, feared that he was easy prey for the street toughs as well as the smooth-talking scam artists. Still, he rebuffed any suggestion that he move.

"If he leaves, to him that means that they ran him away," said his daughter Joyce Greene-Jackson, an administrator with the state Department of Social Services. "He always says, 'I ain't scared of these punks.' And we say, 'Daddy, it's not the same. These people carry guns.' He says, 'They ain't running me away.'"

As a young man Perkins owned a small farm in Dry Branch, Georgia, outside of Macon. He raised chickens and hogs and grew everything from peas to corn to cotton. Dogs had long been part of his life; he always had plenty of hounds around for hunting coon and the like.

In all, Perkins and his wife, Arelia, had seven daughters and four sons. In the late fifties, their oldest sons came to Boston seeking work. The rest of the family followed in 1960.

From the very beginning, home in Boston was a six-room apartment in a three-decker on Intervale Street in Dorchester. To get the flat, Perkins and his wife had to lie about how many kids they had, and they hid a handful of them whenever the landlord showed up. The ruse was soon discovered, though, but rather than kick them out, the owner sold Perkins the place.

It was a safe neighborhood in those days, a section where the kids could play outside or walk down to the ice cream shop after dark without fear.

By the mid-to-late seventies, though, crime and poverty had made inroads on Intervale Street, driving the neighborhood down. It was around that time that Perkins, who had owned a variety of dogs over the years, got wind of a fellow down the street who was moving and could not take his German shepherd with him. Two neighborhood kids brought the dog over for Perkins to inspect. His original name was, of all things, Fido. En route to Perkins's place, the kids, knowing better, dubbed him King.

Perkins gave King, already a full-grown dog, the once-over, fired off some commands, slapping the dog until he obeyed, and decided he would "do the job." He paid twenty-five dollars for him, which turned out to be the bargain of his life.

Immediately, Perkins started training King to be his protector, praising the dog when he complied with his commands and doling out "whuppin's" when he wouldn't. The dog, meanwhile, was never neutered—the very idea made Perkins wince—which only fueled the aggressive side of King's nature. Though Perkins's attitude might have offended a lot of people, he got what he wanted—a loaded gun of a dog. Now he could stroll down any street, King marching free at his side, without a care. The dog stirred wariness in strangers, if not outright fear.

From time to time, Perkins would show King off to his neighbors, sending a less than subtle message that the pair was not to be taken lightly. "My father would play games to show how big and bad King was," remembered Joyce. "He would just stand out there on the street. If anybody went near my father, he would say something like, 'Give me a handshake,' knowing that if the guy made a move toward my father, that King would be all over him. And, of course, the guy wouldn't know what was going on, right? King would be like, 'Arrrrgh! Arrrgh!' And my father would say, 'Yeap, better get back; better not come near me.' And they'd be like, 'All right, Mr. Perkins, all right.'"

Perkins had a guardian all right, but what he may not have expected was the friendship that developed between man and beast. Perkins and his wife separated. With the children gone as well, King was the old man's main companion. Retired now, he took the dog with him everywhere. All around the neighborhood, from the grocery store to the courthouse, everybody knew Tom Perkins and King.

"He was a *man*," said Perkins of his German shepherd. "He didn't play around. He'd do the *job* for *you*. He would do the job for you. He didn't allow nobody in that door. I'd be kinda hot and leave the door open. Nobody come in that door; nobody come in that hallway.

"When I'd go out at night, I'd take him with me. He'd come

up ahead of me and watch and make sure it was safe, then turn around and look back to see if anybody's behind me. If anybody's behind me, they better move, because he's coming back. And he ain't coming back for nothing: take care of some business.

"Gal came to the door one time, knocked on the door, and had a hundred-dollar bill she wanted me to change. I said OK, took out my wallet, and she snatched my wallet and took off. I had about four or five hundred dollars in there. King was back there. If he'd of been up here, she wouldn't have gotten nowhere. I said, 'King!' He knew something was wrong; he flew over here. I said, 'Watch her!' And he went straight to her. He didn't run: he jumped in the air, like one of them wildcats. Jumped right on her back and knocked her down. He held her until I got there and took my money.

"I'll tell you another thing he'd do. If you're sitting here talking, and you say, 'I'm going,' King would go to the door. He wouldn't let you go out that door until you answer to me. I'd say, 'King, let him out; get back.' That's the only way he'd let you go out there.

"That dog was a man. He wouldn't take no joking. I'd been robbed a heap of times if it hadn't been for him. They'd grab something, but they didn't get nowhere. A woman or a man, he didn't care who it was."

One time his daughter Joyce came back to her apartment in another part of town and found she had been robbed. Gone was her television and her new stereo. Though she had no proof, she had strong suspicions that it was a certain neighbor, who she found out was a convicted thief. "I was mad," she remembered, "because everything I had worked hard for was gone. I called my father, and I was crying. Well, what did I do *that* for? My father was like, 'No problem; me and King will be right over.' I said, 'You and King?'

"Well, he came over there with King, and he's yelling about how he's gonna get these people who broke into his daughter's apartment. The people were out, but when they came home, my father opened the door, and there was King standing there."

A tremendous scene ensued, with everyone screaming wildly at each other, and old man Perkins in the middle promising to unleash an all-too-willing King. "Nobody messes with my daughter!" he shouted.

Someone finally summoned the police to calm everyone down, but not before Perkins and King had made an impression. "Those people said, 'Forget this,' and they moved out within a week," said Joyce with a laugh. "It was the fastest move I've ever seen."

Thomas Perkins was indeed full of pride in King's fierce protectiveness, but the dog meant a lot more to him. When Perkins sat in the kitchen chatting with visitors, King made himself comfortable right next to his chair. When he went to bed at night, King settled in nearby. What the old man ate, King ate. As another daughter, Gloria Perkins, put it, "My father didn't feel alone when he had King."

For years Perkins had always left the door to his living room locked. That was his special room, which he kept immaculate, where pictures of his family were displayed, and which he didn't want grandchildren, great-grandchildren, or anyone else to disrupt. "If we had real company from down Georgia, say," said Joyce, "and they wanted to visit my father, we would go sit in the living room, but that would be it—not just everyday people. That was his hands-off room. Nobody was allowed in my father's living room—*Nobody*."

Except, of course, the dog. "King was the exception to every rule," she added. "That was his house and my father's house."

What's more, the dog served to help Perkins get back up to his apartment on days when his hips, wracked by arthritis, were too painful. The old man would lean on the dog for support or hold his collar and have King pull him, step-by-step.

Other times around the apartment, Perkins would stumble, then crash to the floor and find himself unable to rise, or he would lie in bed, too ill to reach the telephone. When that happened King sat at the door barking like mad until the downstairs neighbors came to help.

Perkins may have wanted a bodyguard, but in King he got a lot more. "My father used to say, 'Me and King, we gonna be buried together,'" said Joyce. "'I'm gonna get a plot big enough for me and King.' And I'd tell him, 'We're not gonna bury you with the dog!' He'd say, 'Yes you are!' And I'd say, 'Well, when you go, you won't know, but you will *not* be buried with no dog.'"

Sharing a grave was one thing, but on January 5, 1986, the pair could very well have died together. It was a cloud-covered, freezing Sunday, around six-thirty at night, and Thomas Perkins was watching television when the pounding started on his door.

"Who is it?" he shouted.

"It's me, Uncle Tom," came an unfamiliar voice. "It's me. Open the door."

Perkins cracked the door just a few inches. A black .22-caliber handgun suddenly appeared in his face. "Don't move, old man!" yelled a black man in his early twenties as he shoved the door open. "Give me your money right now! I know you got it!"

King was in another room. Hearing the ruckus, he trotted over, then lunged at the hoodlum, jaws clenching the wrist of his gun hand, according to Perkins. "I thought he was going to shoot," he said, "but King got him before he could pull the trigger. King got that gun down out of my face. He pulled that hand down like a *man*."

The hallway erupted in combat and the gnashing of teeth as the dog drove the intruder against the stairs that led to the third floor. The gunman opened fire, wildly blasting away, striking King four times—twice in the shoulders and twice in his legs.

The gunman broke away from King, burst into the apartment, and staggered into a spare bedroom, locking it behind him. A minute later, though, Perkins opened the door with his key, and the bleeding German shepherd was on the hoodlum again, now more furious than ever, tearing at him, shredding his clothes.

The assailant finally found a moment's reprieve behind a bed. It was around then, however, that Perkins appeared with his shotgun, "Old Bessie," and opened fire. This prompted the invader to make his wisest choice of the day: he went crashing through the window, a two-story free fall to the alley below.

"He didn't get nothin' but his butt kicked and tore up," said Perkins of the intruder. "He thought he was gonna kill King, but King didn't go nowhere. He kept workin' on that nigger; he tore his clothes off of him. When the cops found him, he was tore up and bleeding like a hog. King whupped him like a baby."

But the dog was wounded as well. When the Boston police showed up and saw the bullet holes and blood all over, they tried to detain Perkins for questioning. That was when the old man blew up, telling them to get the hell out of his house. Even injured King managed a growl or two at the lawmen. "I didn't have time for no questions," said Perkins. "My dog was dying."

Or so it seemed. He called Angell Memorial to say he was coming. Though King was bleeding, he managed to walk with Perkins to the car. In fact, the dog clambered right in and settled next to the old man, who never thought twice about the upholstery.

Angell intern Bud Keller, today a veterinary surgeon in Columbia, South Carolina, was on walk-ins that evening. What he found was a dog that had been shot repeatedly at close range but remarkably suffered no life-threatening injuries. The bullets had done damage near each of his shoulders, his left elbow, and his right front foot. No major arteries or organs were pierced. The only fracture was the second toe on his foot, which Keller treated with a bandage and splint. One of the slugs, in King's left shoulder, was never removed, since it was causing no problems. That the rounds were of a small caliber was a blessing.

Years later Dr. Keller was hard pressed to recollect much about Perkins, but he had vivid memories of King. Unlike many injured animals, King was never aggressive or protective of his wounds. "He was a well-behaved, sweet dog," said Keller. "He really was. He would let you handle him with no trouble, even his injured pieces and parts. He would just look at you as if to say, 'Do what you will, I guess you're trying to help me.'"

The Boston papers wrote about the incident, and United Press International followed, spreading the story nationwide. "He's the best friend I ever had," Perkins said of King in one article. "I miss him so much, I'm about to cry." People around the country, touched by King's actions and distressed by his injuries, opened their hearts—and their pocketbooks. Complete strangers sent hundreds of dollars to help defray King's medical expenses. Schoolchildren showered him with get-well cards.

"I come back to get him, and he was all right," Perkins said. "He was glad to see me; he was licking me all in the face. He didn't want nobody around me. And when he come in this house, he come here looking for that guy, trying to find him again. He wanted him again; he would have killed him that time."

The Boston police, however, made an arrest the night of the attack, finding twenty-two-year-old Dennis Bendolph of Roxbury with drug paraphernalia and a fresh bullet wound—of "undetermined origin"—in his left shoulder. Bendolph eventually pleaded guilty to charges of armed robbery on a person over sixty-five, assault, and cruelty to an animal. The judge sentenced him to ten to twelve years in prison.

King, meanwhile, was beloved all the more by the Perkins family. Daughter Joyce, who had always been wary of the dog, now saw him through new eyes. "For some reason I wasn't afraid of him anymore," she said. "To have saved my father's life, King became twice as special to me."

The Shepherd-Dog Club of America named King its hero dog of the year for 1986 and presented him with a handsome silver medal at a ceremony in Rhode Island.

The MSPCA, meanwhile, honored the animal at its first Humane Awards banquet, in 1987, a happy occasion for Perkins and his family. A bronze-colored medal on a green-and-white ribbon was draped around King's neck, and his praises were sung deep into the evening.

The media covered that event as well, and an amusing photograph of the old man offering King a sip from his champagne glass was widely circulated. The *Boston Herald* ran a big picture of a panting King sporting his medal. "Hero pooch fetches award," read the headline. Underneath the picture it read "'ATTA BOY.'"

"I had anything I wanted that night," recalled Perkins, in reverie. "King did, too. King would eat out of the dish with them white ladies. They fed him ice cream, and he'd eat it. I didn't know he would eat ice cream. Boy, they were crazy about King."

A few years passed. Now, just as Perkins was growing old, so too was his dog. Like the old man, King was slow getting from one place to another. Merely rising took longer, and climbing stairs became torturous. "It got to the point where King was just dragging," said Joyce. "He didn't have his pep; he didn't have his speed. My father was dragging. King was dragging. It was kind of sad."

Increasingly, the MSPCA came out to the house to transport King to Angell for one problem or another. Time and again they worked him up, treated him, and shipped him back home.

That last time, though, as shelter worker Amy Knapp drove the animal to the hospital, it seemed clear that he would not return. Veterinarian Alicia Faggella, who examined King that final time, noted that he was struggling to walk. His hind legs crossed over when he tried to move, and it did not take much for him to topple. Faggella's diagnosis was degenerative myelopathy, a deterioration of the spine. The disease was often found in aging German shepherds and other big dogs. There was no cure; it would only get worse.

That day Faggella called Thomas Perkins and explained the situation. It was time, she said, to consider euthanasia.

Perkins was heartbroken, but he understood. "If you have to, go ahead," he said. "Just don't tell me about it."

At ten after six that evening, one good dog, as much a hero as any animal could be, was put out of his misery. If someone had thought of it, perhaps the MSPCA would have arranged for a special plot and headstone for King at the society's pet cemetery in Methuen, Massachusetts. As it was, he was cremated with a lot of other dead dogs and cats, perhaps heroes in their own rights, their ashes anonymously buried.

A few years later, Thomas Perkins still mourned his loss. Since King's death he had owned other dogs, but none worked out. "He keeps trying to find a King, but he can't find a King," said Joyce. "He's had a lot of dogs—a lot. He'll tell me every now and then, 'You know, I'll never have another dog like King. This dog here, he's not like King.' And I'll say, 'Yeah, Daddy, I know: he's not like King.'

"When King had to be put to sleep, I'm telling you, a part of my father died and never came back."

Down on Intervale Street, Thomas Perkins would be inclined to agree. He had owned plenty of dogs in his life, but it had taken seven decades to find a trueheart. "That was a wonderful dog," Perkins said one late summer morning, situated at his kitchen table, the ghost of King at his feet. "Never been a dog in the world like him, and there never will be again.

"Yeah, poor boy had to go. I've got to go, too, one day. All of us have to go; we didn't come here to stay.

"I hope King's in heaven today, waiting for me, because I'll be there one day with him."

PART FIVE *Sanctuary*

Look homeward Angel now, and melt with ruth.

—JOHN MILTON, "Lycidas"

21

Change

THEY LOOKED LIKE THEY BELONGED IN A SURREALISTIC painting: a dozen men and women, dressed like the professionals that they were, heads bowed, each solitarily studying the floor at different points along a dusky stretch of corridor. Most wore small grins.

It was seven-thirty in the morning. What had captured the attention of the veterinarians and staff, beginning a new week, was a path of computer paper—scrawled upon in multiple colors and taped to the floor with white bandage tape—that ran the entire forty to fifty yards of hallway.

For hospital personnel only, this hall stretched from a wooden door just beyond the front office and continued past the business department, the intern Hole, the offices of Doug Brum and a few other veterinarians, and ended at the library. This was the same route, coincidence of coincidences, that the incoming class of interns would take to get to this morning's orientation meeting with Brum and Paul Gambardella. Smiling faces would not be what first welcomed these young veterinarians to their new jobs and a new city; instead, they would be met by the Walk of Terror—courtesy, of course, of the out-going interns, who would depart from Angell in a month.

All morning they came and went to read the dozens of messages along the paper trail: staff doctors, office workers, techs, nurses. And, of course, the new interns, looking so much more green, and sober, than anyone else around as they read their way along the brown-tiled floor toward their first meeting as employees at Angell Memorial Animal Hospital.

"Welcome new interns. Suckers. Danger."

"Do you know how to unblock a cat? You will in a week."

"Notice that there are no windows in the interns' office. They know if you see outside you will leave."

"If you treasure your life . . . you should turn around right now."

A woman from the financial office shook her head. "Do you see what they do to these people?" she asked. "They're awful. The problem is that they can still run out that door—"

"I'm thinking about it," said one of the rookies, standing nearby.

"—and leave *us* holding the bag."

Jittery when they arrived, some of the new interns were now wide-eyed. Some nervously chuckled. One or two laughed louder than their first-day status dictated. Most did not skip a single word.

"It's not worth aging 25 years for this. You'll find more white hairs in your head than you can pluck."

"You'll love those referral *dumps* on Friday and Saturday night. And weekends at Angell."

"Could a domestic cat kill a human being? Yes!"

Halfway down the hall, leashes dangled from a rafter in the style of nooses.

"Forget about the sun. . . . You'll never see it."

"Forget about the moon. You won't see it either."

One of the liaisons read a few samples and moved on. "It's a shame," she said, "that this is the only time that they do such intricate paperwork."

"Say good-bye to life's pleasures. No Fun. No dates. No sex. No nothing."

"Be prepared for shit rolling downhill . . . because *you* are at the bottom."

"Are you SCARED about your first overnight? Don't worry...if you only kill 5 or 6 things it will be okay."

"This is your last chance to run!"

"Welcome to Angell's concentration camp. You can walk in . . . but you'll *never* walk out."

"If you walk through this door, you're doomed."

"*Don't* do it. *No* sex for one year. It's not too late."

More leash nooses hung from the library entrance.

"This is the *Final Countdown*. You're about to blow up and become an insignificant particle in our vast cosmos."

There was a cartoon bomb, the typical ball with fuse alight. And then a countdown: "Ten," "nine," "eight," . . . on into the library, where the final message was a single word:

"BOOM!"

The outgoing interns had stayed up half the night, preparing what had become an annual tradition, this paper pathway of forewarning and advice for their successors. In the process, some took potshots at members of the staff. There were personal slaps thinly disguised as jokes for everyone to read about specific doctors and even entire departments.

Some feelings were hurt that Monday morning, but none took as much umbrage as the intensive care nurses. "Let me tell you about the ICU nurses," one of the interns had written on the Carpet of Freedom. "Did you ever really hate someone?" And then: "Who will be the first to get in a fight with Joan?" The reference was to ICU nurse Joan Fontaine.

As in human hospitals, Angell had tensions between its nurses and doctors. Usually they revolved around patient care, but personality conflicts and the workplace hierarchy played parts as well. Tensions were most evident with the interns, who were about the same age as many of the nurses. The young doctors showed up at Angell ranked among the highest in their veterinary school classes, often with prestigious college pedigrees. But they were inexperienced. The nurses, on the other hand, came from a variety of backgrounds, and a number of them lacked even a bachelor's degree. Still, they were trained, watchful, and tended to know the nature of the animals under their care, often better than the veterinarians. Most of them had been around the hospital a while, some for many years.

So when some babyface from Penn State or Cornell or Cal–Davis rolled in, as they did every year, and started ordering questionable dosages or dubious medications, the nurses called them on it. When an intern resorted to shouts of "I am the doctor; you are the nurse!" a few of the nurses threw it back in their face. If push came to shove, the nurses simply called in the veterinarian in charge of ICU and showed her the medical records. If the orders were in fact off, God save the mariner.

On the other hand, the nurses were not always right. Some interns felt the remarks and questions were tactics to undermine them and put them in their place. A lot of the nurses had inserted hundreds of IVs into thread-thin veins and could do it effortlessly. They knew the treatments that Angell's doctors used in certain situations. Someone fresh out of vet school, though, usually needed a minute to perform basic tasks. Often, too, they had learned new or different approaches to various medical problems. It was frustrating to have a nurse jump on you over such matters.

What's more, the starting pay for most of the nurses was close to eight dollars an hour, with breaks and a union contract to boot. Some of the interns calculated that their own wages came to about a dollar sixty-five an hour. They came to Angell for experience, not money, but it could still be a sore point.

It got so bad in years past that certain nurses refused to defer to interns by using the title "doctor." Even now there were moments when a confused intern would turn to a nurse for advice and hear in reply, "You're the *'doctor'*."

Both sides had their points. Some interns were self-confident beyond their abilities and needed what nurse Fontaine called "reality therapy." The nurses, however, were not above one-upmanship. Seniority, they figured, had its privileges.

Most notorious of the nurses was Fontaine, who, in her mid-thirties, had been at Angell for more than ten years. She was named after the movie star but was otherwise unrelated. Fontaine had a BS in wildlife biology, was a licensed emergency medical technician, and followed both veterinary and human medical journals. Her goal was to someday work as an emergency room physician.

Fontaine worked in intensive care full-time, while the others on her shift rotated in and out from the general wards. She complained often about Angell politics. Still, she knew her work and used sarcasm to rebuff those she thought didn't know theirs. "I wouldn't trust him with my pet rock" was Joan's trademark jibe at certain veterinarians. She dubbed one intern "the Doorstop," "because that's all she's good for." And when a client told Fontaine, in a patronizing tone, that he was an M.D., she rolled her eyes. "Your mother must be very proud," she said dryly.

"My reason for being here is to take care of the patients," Joan said. "I'm not here to stroke anyone's ego, least of all a DVM's. I've got a job to do, and it's gonna get done. If I happen to stomp all over your inflated ego, then you leave it outside of ICU with your coffee."

Now, with the interns apparently saying they *hated* them, the nurses in intensive care were both wounded and seething. Most of them had gotten along well with this group. They were furious the interns would publicly post a remark like that. "It ticks you off," said one, "when you think we're all just trying to do the best for the animals."

"They think they're the only ones who do any work around here," said another. "Except Lynne Morris." She pointed to what was in fact Morris's handwriting amidst all the other inscriptions. "Listen to the ICU nurses," Morris has scrawled. "They do know stuff!!"

"What the nurses have to realize," said their supervisor, Susan Fernandes, "is that as they work here year after year, they mature— the interns don't." In other words, new interns arrived each June, ready to make the same mistakes and, at times, behave as sophomoric as those before them. Forever and ever, world without end. Sometimes the youthful energy invigorated the staff. Sometimes it got old quickly.

By midday someone removed the offending passages, leaving a

conspicuous gap in the paper trail. In ICU, meanwhile, the outgoing interns were feeling a chill in the air.

Not from Joan Fontaine, however. In fact, she laughed out loud when she saw her name on the Walk of Fame. Joan adored a good rhubarb and was ready to jump in on a moment's notice. "It's like I was saying yesterday," she told a fellow nurse. "'I can't wait for the new interns to get here. They can't be any worse than these idiots.'"

MOST OF THE NEW INTERNS AS WELL AS BRUM AND Gambardella, found seats around some pushed-together tables in the Angell Memorial library to begin orientation. A handful more were en route to Boston from points west.

Originally, the computerized match had given Angell ten paid interns, all women. But soon after, Gambardella was able to add four more, two who happened to be men and three of whom would work without pay. Now nine women and one of the men were at the table, dressed for the first time in white coats as honest-to-God veterinarians. They were proud of that, but apprehensive.

Gambardella, who spoke first, was not exactly Knute Rockne. He simply told his new charges what they could expect. For the next month, he explained, each intern would be assigned a member of the outgoing class to follow and learn the ropes from. Sometime by July 15, when the previous class graduated, the newcomers would know enough to take on their own cases.

It was, as the Walk of Terror hinted, a scary proposition. In most other programs the interns had less of a burden. Cases were usually assigned to a "service," meaning staff doctors essentially made the calls and the interns carried out the orders.

At Angell permanent staff doctors did look over most patients, usually on rounds, and were available for advice. But unless an intern's treatment plan was way out of line, the case was in the hands of the intern alone. This unsettled some clients to the point of white-hot rage. "You're a farmer," one had written to one intern in an invective-filled letter that spring, "not a doctor."

At the same time, people often blamed interns for no other reason than their being young. Hospital officials felt strongly that their system of checks and balances was as adequate as it could be without eviscerating the very heart of the internship. Most of the young doctors, they pointed out, acquitted themselves well. All of them became veterans quick.

"Big-city clients can be demanding," Gambardella now told them, "but this hospital is in a fishbowl. Everybody is watching you—the public, the nurses, the outside veterinarians. You'll see everything once, and, of course, the routine things you'll see a lot of. By the time you leave, you'll have a firm foundation not only in medicine and surgery, but how to deal with clients. People skills, unfortunately, come from the school of hard knocks."

Doug Brum pulled up a cardboard box and from it gave them their name tags, bandage scissors, formularies, keys, locker assignments, MSPCA packets, and guides to Boston. Still treasuring his own intern days, Brum tried to explain how the interns could make the most of it. He liked people who wanted to learn, who were willing to take on new or potentially difficult situations.

He also wanted them to understand how important it was simply to get along. "There's a real spirit to the internship, and it's different than most, because you guys have a lot of responsibility and you're out there alone," he said. "When things are bad, when it's real busy, you need each other. If one person has fourteen in and someone else has one in, the guy with one should help out. That's the key to the internship and the key to enjoying it."

It also should not be Us Against Them. What made it all come together was working within the bigger scheme of Angell, be it with the liaisons or the front office staff or the staff doctors. It mattered, he said, how you handled people. "There's always potential tension between the lay staff and the new vets coming in because the lay staff is good," Brum said. "They are. But they're not vets. They're not new vets, either. You guys know a lot of things they don't.

"Let's take ICU nurses, for example. They're *really* good. I still learn stuff from them every day. I go in and I SOAP my cases (evaluate patients by means of Subjective, Objective Assessment Plans) in the morning, then I come back maybe at five or six and look at the case again. The nurses are in there the whole day with that case. Some of them have been doing it for ten years. If they call me in the middle of the day, and they say this dog doesn't look quite right, I don't blow them off. I trust them. If I go back and I say, 'Aw, he looks fine; he's just hungry,' I also say, 'Hey, thanks for letting me know, but I think we're OK here. Let me know if it changes.'

"Work with them. They can be your major ally or a major headache. If your attitude is, 'This is the way it is, this is the way it's gonna be, and that's it, it's gonna be a problem—for both of you. You're not gonna gain their help. And they've got a lot to give you.

"Just learn to use them and trust them."

BY THE END OF DAY ONE, MOST OF THE NEW INTERNS would be swimming in information. They learned of bladder rounds, in which the late-night intern was responsible for squeezing empty the bladders of patients that would not urinate on their own. They found where to check for their messages each morning, where to sign in, and where to write the name of every animal that was euthanized or died in-house. They were warned of whose handwriting was awful. Not a few people suggested that for their own survival they be nice to the ICU nurses.

Tim Becker, one of the new arrivals, discovered that he would be the first to serve overnight duty. As a prank the outgoing intern who would handle all the cases that night and teach Becker the ropes called in sick. Brum played along, telling Becker what "happened" and asking whether he was up to caring for everything in the hospital, plus every new disaster that came in the door, by his lonesome.

Becker, ranked first in his veterinary school class at Tufts, was ready for a lot of thrills at Angell. But not this, not so soon. He looked like his physician had just told him that his test came back positive, and no, there was no cure.

"Well," Becker finally stammered, "I don't know where all the things are. And, uh, well, I guess I can do it. Sure, I can do it. Better sooner than later."

Everyone broke out laughing.

That day, too, a client happened to ask new intern Leslie Schwarz, who had been tagging along with one of the outgoing interns, whether she was a student or a doctor. Fresh out of the University of Missouri, the intern started to answer "Student," when it dawned on her: "No," she told the woman, "I'm a doctor."

That in itself felt pretty good.

IT WAS TUESDAY, THE DAY AFTER, WHEN THE BIG bouquet of flowers arrived for the intensive care nurses. Joan Fontaine pointed with her thumb down the hall to the nurse's station where they were displayed, smiled sardonically, and murmured something about the interns doing penance.

"We love you," read the message on the card. It was signed, "The interns." Angell could now march onward, with one less dispute, one bundle of bad feelings mollified.

The interns, though, had never purchased those please-forgive-us flowers. It was Doug Brum.

22

Fontaine

BACK IN THE SPRING, JOAN FONTAINE HAD BEEN OUT in her pickup truck, her dog Duke sitting at her side. She slowed to stop at a red light, and a strange sorrow washed over her. Something was telling her that Duke, a sturdy brown cross between a Doberman pinscher and a German shepherd, was soon to die.

Fontaine was thin, with short, blonde hair and long, mischievous features. She drew serious as she wondered what would cause the death of this dog that she had owned for thirteen years. Inexplicably, she ran a hand across his belly. "Is this how you're going to die?" she asked.

Into the summer this sense of foreboding pursued her: something was going to kill Duke, and whatever it was would be in his stomach. As it was, the animal showed few symptoms of disease. He vomited maybe once a month these past six months—unusual, but nothing of major concern. On her regular runs with him, Joan also noticed that Duke had slowed down some. Given his age, that was no surprise either.

Early in the summer Fontaine brought him in for a workup, just to be sure. At that time veterinarian Alicia Faggella discovered a heart murmur but said it was mainly just something to keep in mind. Most everything else seemed fine.

Duke had been Fontaine's pet for the better part of her adulthood. She adopted him not long after starting at Angell as a ward attendant. He had entered the hospital with a broken leg after dog met car on the streets of Dorchester. The people who brought him in said they were the owners but never returned. So when Duke, then only six or seven months old, finally made the short list of unwanted dogs to be euthanized, Fontaine said what the hell, she would take him.

For her trouble, she got a dog that needed to learn some manners; he lapped his tongue at everything in sight when the refrigerator door was open and tried to scarf food right off of counters. She liked, though, how a section of fur on his back ran counter to his overall coat, giving him the exotic look of a Rhodesian Ridgeback. As time passed she also found the dog to be a reliable running partner, fearsome guardian, and friend.

Duke, whom Joan nicknamed Caribou, had been healthy, too. When the weather turned cold or rainy, he limped some, the result of his old injury. But in all those years, he never spent another night at Angell because of illness.

Then one day in August, Duke wouldn't eat. Joan finally offered him some food from her hand, and he nibbled a little. The next day he seemed better, eating as usual and running with Joan about a mile. One day later, though, he ignored his food again. He was breathing heavily, too. This time when Fontaine brought her fingers to his belly, she could feel a slight wave of fluid just beneath the body wall.

That afternoon she was on a hospital telephone, calling Doug Brum, whom she had to track down in the labyrinth that was Angell. "Hi, is this my dog's doctor?" Brum had known Fontaine for years, since his internship. Sometimes she drove him crazy with her cynicism, a trait that he lacked. Still, he liked joking with her and considered her the best nurse in the place. Her regular veterinarian, Faggella, was off all week, so she came to Doug. It was something of a distinction, given how critical Joan was about so many of Angell's veterinarians.

"Hi, Joan," Brum said. "What's up?"

"Well, Duke hasn't been eating very well for the past couple of days, and I get a hint that he may have some abdominal distension. He's got a belly full of blood. I think he's got an abdominal tumor."

Brum smirked. Gallows humor was the order of the day at Camp Angell, and no one played the game any better than Fontaine. "Yeah, right," he said. "Now, what's up?"

"Doug, my dog's bleeding to his abdomen. He is."

Brum came and looked Duke over in an examination room. He too could feel the fluid wave, but no unusual mass. He ordered blood work and radiographs. The dog's liver enzymes were slightly elevated, possibly a sign of trouble. On the X rays, the liver looked larger than normal, and a cloudiness across parts of the film suggested fluid in the abdomen and chest.

When Brum went to tap the fluid, he knew it was bad. Joan's face grew wan, not at the sight of the pure blood that came out, but at the likelihood that her dire predictions were on target.

It would turn out that Duke's platelet count was way down. The dog, in fact, was low-grade DIC (disseminated intravascular coagulation), a clotting abnormality that results in internal bleeding and often signals cancer. Roundly, DIC is also said to stand for "death is coming."

Brum could not say for sure, but the signs were pointing to hemangiosarcoma, an aggressive cancer often seen in German shepherds, among other breeds. It was difficult to treat, especially when it struck vital organs. An ultrasound strengthened Doug's belief that it was in the liver, though perhaps the pancreas.

No one had to tell Fontaine about cancer's ravaging effects. In the mid-1980s, her older sister, Beverly, had died of ovarian cancer a harrowing fourteen months after diagnosis. She was forty-five years old, a science teacher, with a husband and three kids. Of her three sisters and two brothers, Joan had been closest to Bev, who was sixteen years older and practically a second mother. Even with the passage of years, Bev's death was a tender place beneath Fontaine's thick skin. "I really loved my sister," she said simply.

If any good came of the experience, it was that Joan learned a lot about cancer. She became a clearinghouse of information for a number of coworkers whose family members had been stricken by the disease. Joan understood that death from cancer could be torturous. Euthanasia, she felt, was one area in which the veterinary field had a step up on human medicine. Because they had that option, owners and veterinarians made Joan angry when they went to outlandish lengths to save animals that had obviously reached the end of the line. "That's life and death in the big city," Fontaine said earlier in the summer. "Nobody's gonna get out of this world alive. And that includes your pet."

Once she even told a client, tongue in cheek, that if she wanted an animal companion that would live longer than herself, the lady should look into a tortoise. That was the Joan that most people around the hospital knew: wisecracking, matter-of-fact, streetwise. Even now when she went to take her ailing dog for a brief walk outside, it was the same routine. "Come on," she said, "let's take a piss."

Doug Brum, however, knew she was hurting. He noticed that her eyes were brimmed red from crying and lack of sleep. He watched how she stroked Duke's coat and talked softly to him, like one might to a child. The bond was obvious.

For his part, Brum liked that so many of his coworkers turned to him as their veterinarian. At the same time, he hated having to see someone like Joan so exposed. It was difficult, as well as emotionally draining, to see a friend in pain. "It absolutely sucks," was how Brum phrased it.

On Friday, after two nights in the hospital, Duke was scheduled for exploratory surgery. One of the nurses brought in her own dog as a blood donor. Duke would need fresh blood to help combat the complications that could arise in surgery from the clotting abnormality. Odds were small that the surgeon would discover an easily remedied problem. Joan decided that if it was hemangiosarcoma and it was pervasive, she would order that Duke be euthanized right on the table to spare him inevitable suffering.

That afternoon, as the techs were about to take Duke to be anesthetized and prepped for surgery, Joan went over to him in the hall. She ran her hand along his fur and spoke quietly. "Look, if I don't see you again, Bev's gonna take care of you until I do."

JOAN ELIZABETH FONTAINE GREW UP IN MEDFORD, a blue-collar town just north of Boston. Her father was a pressman in the graphic arts department at the Massachusetts Institute of Technology, and her mother a medical secretary. Hollywood's Joan Fontaine had always been one of her mother's favorite actresses. She had long toyed with the idea of naming one of the kids after her, so when the last one came along and it was a girl, Joan Fontaine she became.

With six children crashing around the house, Joan being the youngest, it was no wonder she became a scrapper. It took little to ignite a battle royal amongst the Fontaine siblings. "I remember having fistfights with my brother over who was gonna eat the last of the spinach," Joan said.

The Fontaine household was a wildlife sanctuary of its own design, as the kids offered refuge to everything from nomadic dogs to injured squirrels. One time Joan and her sister hid a stray dog in the garage, fearing that her parents would make them get rid of it. The kids snuck it food, but then the weather turned cold. Joan refused to leave the animal's side, despite her father's repeated calls to come inside for the night. "Get in here!" he finally yelled.

"No!" Joan shouted, bursting into tears. "I don't want to leave the dog!"

"The dog! What dog?"

"The one that's been in the garage for a week!"

In the summer the family vacationed at a cottage her father had built in Plymouth. Her brothers would hunt bullfrogs with a BB gun and use them for bait. Young Joan rescued the ones she could, removed the BBs with tweezers, then attempted to sew the frogs back up. "They never survived surgery, though," she remembered with a shrug.

"And then we had a little hill of sand that we called Boot Hill. Any roadkill we found or animal that didn't make it, we'd build a little casket for him and bury him."

Fontaine saw herself as the protector of smaller and weaker kids in her neighborhood. Even as an adult, she relished the memory of bloodying an older kid's nose for hurting one of her sisters. "I saw him later," Joan said. "His mother was dragging him into the house. He had his nose all taped up. I'm like, 'Go ahead, you little bastid; come back again, and I'll nail ya!'" She was four.

All of her brothers and sisters were academic achievers and went on to successful careers in the sciences. Joan followed her heart into wildlife biology at the University of Massachusetts–Amherst. She also developed an interest in emergency medical work and earned her state and national certifications.

After graduation Fontaine took a job at Angell, intending to eventually go into wildlife disease biology, possibly as a veterinarian. Soon she entered the training program and became a nurse—good experience, she figured, for when she applied to veterinary school.

At Angell the intensive care unit doubled as an emergency room. Fontaine was able to combine her interest in animals with her passion for emergency medical work. Now, however, she was working with trauma victims, albeit animals, of all kinds. There were stabbings, shootings, chokings, poisonings, and, of course, those that had been hit by cars. It was exciting. She learned a lot. Her plans of being a wildlife biologist soon fell away.

Fontaine also found her Angell experience more rewarding than her other career interest of becoming an emergency medical technician. At one point she even turned down an opportunity at a full-time job. "As an EMT, the only drug you can give is oxygen," she said. "At Angell I was learning a lot more technical skills. I can put catheters in something that is less than a pound up to something that's two hundred and fifty pounds. I've put chest tubes in all sorts of stuff. And I learned a lot about medicine, the way a diabetic patient is treated or a cardiac patient."

Joan became one of the hospital's top nurses, now earning

about three hundred thirty dollars a week, but she had reached as far as she could in patient care without a veterinary school degree. Her sister's illness and time spent visiting her in the hospital, meanwhile, sparked an interest in human medicine. She directed herself toward someday working as an emergency room physician, though she was rejected in her initial efforts to enter medical school.

Her talents and personality, though, made Fontaine one of the few non-veterinarians to be known across the entire hospital. When a client or staffer was in sudden medical distress, most people knew to seek out Joan.

Many also knew of her sarcasm and varied misadventures. One time a nun was in the waiting room for a checkup of her black Labrador retriever, whose personality seemed to be changing. Fontaine was walking by them, leaving the building, when the dog lunged forward and sunk its teeth into her thigh.

"Jesus fucking Christ!" screamed Joan, clinging to the woodwork, as the animal was pried away.

Later, word came back from the semi-informed front office that Joan should watch her mouth: there was, after all, a nun in the building today. And when a supervisor filling out an accident report routinely inquired how such an incident could be prevented in the future, Fontaine looked askance at him. "Gee, I don't know," she said. "I guess I'll leave the building through a window from now on."

Fontaine had a reputation as one of Angell's premier malcontents. She saw what she regarded as the hospital's flaws and always spoke her mind. Nowadays, she complained often about "the old boys' club" that ran the society and the hospital. She dubbed Paul Gambardella "Little Big Man." She pointed out that no senior veterinarian then on staff was female. She regarded certain veterinarians as incompetents. And, she found it maddening that MSPCA donations might be spent to furnish some bigwig's office upstairs while the wards went without cat pans.

On any given day, Fontaine could be found on duty in intensive care, wearing the aqua green scrubs that were the uniforms of the nurses. Joan usually wore a long-sleeved T-shirt underneath, with a handy hemostat clipped to the bottom of her scrub-shirt pocket. On breaks, she wandered up to the second-floor cafeteria, carrying a hand scanner that monitored local emergency calls. She liked to tune in on these real-life dramas, gleaning bits and pieces of protocol that she hadn't known, as well as hearing the names and voices of her EMT friends.

Joan could be caustic, but those who got to know her saw another side to her personality. Alicia Faggella, who headed ICU, said she had seen Fontaine more than once going beyond the call of duty, sprucing up the unit and making sure everything was perfect in preparation for a television or film crew's arrival. "No matter how much she complains," Faggella said, "she has a very big loyalty to this place."

Her fellow nurses thought highly of her, too. When one discovered Joan staying late one day to feed some animals, the woman scolded her: "You better leave now, or people are going to think you're a nice person."

One elderly man, who spoke to her often during the weeks that his pet was in the unit, exclaimed to me one day, "That Joan is some woman!" Fontaine had taken up a collection to buy his dog a special, comfortable pad to sleep on.

When Fontaine got home—she lived with her parents—she liked to run a few miles with Duke, study for one class or another that she was always taking, or switch on the TV. She didn't gravitate toward "American Gladiators" or professional wrestling, as one might guess, but "Oprah."

Once I told her that I got a kick out of the talk shows in which the wife, girlfriend, and audience all came down on some hapless philanderer. "The ones I like," she replied, "are the reunions of lost loved ones."

A BLUE-CLAD TECH POKED HER HEAD INTO STERILE surgery, which was busy with the final operations of the week. Rock music wafted from the radio, punctuated by the incessant beeps of heart monitors up and down the row of operating tables. "Exploratory's ready!"

"OK, let's have him," said Rose Henle, the supervisor. She went over and grabbed the gurney carrying Duke, who was unconscious, his underside shaved to the skin. Rose wheeled him over and slid him from gurney to operating table in one smooth motion.

Rose was spreading yellowish betadyne, an antiseptic, onto his heaven-facing belly when a coworker happened to glance at the paperwork.

"This is Joan Fontaine's dog," she said, surprised.

Rose paused for a second, eyes widening above her surgical mask. She hadn't known either. "Hmmmm—we don't want anything to happen to him, now, do we?" she asked with a naughty laugh.

The coworker strode away, saying, "I want nothing to do with that dog—noth-ing. I don't want Joan to run me over with her truck. If something went wrong and she saw me on the street, she'd run me over, stop, then back over me."

Fontaine had asked Barbara Gores, a resident from Tufts, to be Duke's surgeon. Gores was talented, but she had years less experience than any of the staff surgeons. Yet she was someone with whom Fontaine felt comfortable, who struck Joan as more than a cutter. Too many surgeons, Fontaine believed, cared only about their immediate handiwork—the sturdiness of the repaired bone, the clean removal of tumor—and not the overall condition of patients. "Common sense has been bred out of the human species," she said one time, "and surgeons are the prime, A–number one examples of it."

Gores was apprehensive. Fontaine's reputation preceded her. What's more, Duke's illness had the potential to be a drawn-out, complicated ordeal. If the animal's problem was sufficiently bad, Gores guessed that Joan might have Duke euthanized. On the other hand, if it was something operable but still not easily corrected, treatment could continue for months, at great expense, without any guarantee of recovery.

When Gores had sliced open the dog's midsection stem to stern, Doug Brum came into sterile surgery. His head was covered with a mask and a surgical cap; a blue gown cloaked his street clothes.

Together they surveyed the scene. Most of the organs looked normal. As Brum had expected, the liver was the source of the problem. A deep red, it was spotted with purplish reddish growths, some the size of coins, but one on the left side as big as a man's fist. "Leever," said Brum in a strange, foreign accent to an intern who had stopped to watch. "Lumps and bumps all over the leever."

One by one, Gores sliced away several slivers of tumor, setting them on a cloth to the side for Brum. When he had all he needed, Brum grabbed the samples and paperwork and hurried out the exit. "OK," he said, "I'm going down." While Gores—and Duke's innards—waited, Brum hurried through Angell's halls and down the stairs to pathology, where Jim Carpenter and his team were finishing their week's work.

Because time was of the essence, everything went on hold in pathology when a doctor came in with a rush surgical sample. Even on short notice, Carpenter's staff could prepare slides for analysis in only five or ten minutes. Though not of the same quality of slides that have more time to set, they were usually good enough to identify most lesions. Good enough, usually, for the veterinarian, surgeon, and patient's owner to come to a decision on what to do next.

At the five-headed microscope, there was little doubt that this was anything good. The first slide, a sample from one of the tumor surfaces, was inconclusive. "Boy, there's so much blood here," Carpenter said. "It does make you worry about hemangiosarcoma, but I can't diagnose it based on what I see. Maybe it's a big blood clot."

The next slide was more definitive. "High power," said Carpenter, informing his resident, Joe McCoy, of the microscope setting. "Oval. Round. Large. Spindle cells. The cells I'm pointing to are greatly compatible with hemangiosarcoma."

The third slide clinched it. "Oh, boy," said Carpenter. "Look at the nuclei there. The size and different shapes. You've got a round one. You've got a linear one. This is a beautiful slide . . ."

Hemangiosarcoma.

The pathologist raised his head from the microscope and looked across to McCoy. "Joe? Do you agree with the diagnosis?"

"Yes, I do."

Brum thanked everyone and hustled back upstairs. He rushed through dirty surgery. "Barb!" he shouted. "Tell Barb it's hemangio! I'm gonna talk to Joan."

Brum found her sitting back in radiology with some friends from her shift, their workday now over. "How does it look?" Joan asked when Brum came in.

He crouched next to her chair, leaned in, and softly explained that it was in fact hemangiosarcoma. There was, he said, a mass the size of a baseball.

"Is it resectable?"

Brum shook his head: not unless Duke came with spare parts. The cancer seemed to affect all of the liver.

"Put him down," said Joan. She paused for a moment. "Make it a hospital disposal." In other words, she had no wish for the remains. Brum went to prepare a syringe of euthanasia solution, then passed it inside for Gores.

Next he went back to Fontaine, who was still with her friends, doing her best to keep the atmosphere as what-the-hellish as possible. She asked for recommendations for a dog that promised never to break a human heart. "What kind of dog doesn't have disease? What's the safest one? A Chihuahua?"

Brum grinned. "No," he said, "you have to get a mix. You should get something really mean, that bites, that you don't like anyway. Then you won't care when it dies."

They talked a little more, never saying much more about Duke or the surgery. Brum went to leave. But as he did, he found he could no longer endure Fontaine's hard-guy routine. He wrapped his arms around her and hugged. "Hell," he would later say, "I did that for myself."

23

Challenge

IT HAD NOT BEEN THE BEST OF YEARS FOR PAUL Gambardella.

At the close of each month, Angell's updated caseload statistics landed on his desk, and the news was seldom good. Time after time the numbers revealed a drop in patient visits to the tune of almost 6.5 percent. By year's end the hospital would have seen 41,381 patients, 3,000 fewer than the year before. Income from clients would tumble from $6.39 million to $6.15 million—and that was with a hefty 8-percent increase in fees.

Competition was the main reason for the decline, Paul felt. As Tufts and other veterinary schools turned out more and more specialists, Angell was weakened. New doctors were opening practices, claiming referrals that once would have come through Angell's doors. Tufts itself, though thirty miles away, was also taking away potential income.

Gambardella also felt that Angell's staff simply had to provide better service. Too many complaints had been made about surly help. The veterinarians, of all people, had to communicate better with the outside veterinarians who referred cases and, by all means, the clients. The staff in the liaison's office still chuckled guiltily when they recalled overhearing one doctor on the telephone trying to explain to an out-of-touch client that her dog was dying: "What I'm trying to say, ma'am," he snapped, "is don't go out and buy any more dog food."

To Paul, who had been given a mandate to rein in the hospital's finances, the budget was a low-level disaster. In previous years Gambardella and his department heads had launched an all-out assault on expenses, cutting back on overtime pay and whatever other costs they could spare. They avoided layoffs, but when low-level staff left the hospital, they were usually not replaced.

Now, not much was left to cut. Gambardella wondered whether at some point he would have to lay off a veterinarian or two, which would be unprecedented at the hospital. In the long run, with fewer people to do the work, such a move could threaten the caseload even further. "When I let a veterinarian go I also let go of all the goddamn gross income they make," Gambardella said, "and I let go of a service they provide. And who's going to do that service? The people that are left behind?"

Still, income was down. Paul figured he could wrangle his way through one or two more years of trouble, but sooner or later something had to give. "The grocery store does it," he said of layoffs. "The hardware store does it. Why can't we?" Paul worried. The budget itself kept him awake nights. And when he got up in the morning, it was still churning in his mind.

Added to the mix was the endless stream of client complaints—some legitimate, some debatable, and some outlandish—that ate up the hours at work. Worst were the confrontations and the insults. One letter writer began, "Dr. Gambardella—You are gross and lower than a snake's belly. How dare you turn my account over to a credit agency after the shitty care my poor dog got on his last visit to your greedy hospital." Another likened him to "smegma."

It was not too hard to dismiss the professional complainers and crazies, but sometimes clients were damn right to be mad. While

Gambardella had no direct involvement in the wrong dog's being opened up in surgery once, it was he who bore the brunt of the owner's rage. Such burdens came with the job, but even that knowledge didn't make it any easier.

From time to time, Paul debated leaving Angell for private practice, or at least going to President Thornton to ask to be relieved of his duties as chief of staff and returned to surgery, even if only for three days a week. "The biggest thing is that I'm not having fun anymore," he said at one particularly trying point. "Every day, it seems, there's another major confrontation that I have to deal with."

Still, he remained. His energy ebbed and flowed, but as the year edged toward a close, he felt a strong will to press on. For one thing, various schemes to increase revenues were finally taking shape. A satellite operation was planned for suburban Lexington, where it was hoped that Angell specialists would draw clients from the upscale suburbs. The preventive medicine Wellness Program was now in place, too. The idea was to better educate clients about basic care of their pets, so as to avoid more serious problems down the line.

Gambardella had a lot invested in the hoped-for success of these changes. On the one hand, it would protect his job. "This office has only one exit," he said. "My neck is on the line here." On the other, it would allow him to spend more time putting together broken animals instead of shuffling papers and sitting in meetings.

Some, however, believed that this was a battle Gambardella would never win. "I would like to do more surgery," he told me. "I really would. And I think there's a way of doing that. If we can get all these programs to run smoothly, if we can get a handle on whatever it is that's keeping us from having forty-four thousand cases a year again, and if we can get that line out the door again—so that I don't have to worry about numbers—then all we have to do is fine-tune the management. And then *I'm* gonna be needed less up here."

At least that was his dream.

24
Gone Fishing

THE BAIT STORES WERE CLOSED FOR THE LABOR DAY weekend, so Jim Carpenter brought along what worms he could uncover, some hotdogs, and a chunk of cheese to whet the fish's appetites.

The pathologist and I were floating along the glassy surface of the Charles River west of Boston in a thirty-year-old aluminum fishing boat that Carpenter had inherited from his father. The two-horse-power outboard was silent, the only sounds being the buzz of insects, the whirr of our reels casting, and the plunk of hotdog on water.

These days Carpenter was taking more time for himself, his reward for more than three decades of labor. He had a vacation to Wisconsin scheduled, was planning a hunting trip in Canada with brother Doug, and by the end of the year would treat himself to an expensive new double-barrel shotgun, "the Cadillac of all guns," as he put it.

On short notice, though, fishing was the pathologist's favorite form of relaxation. Today he dressed in baggy jeans, a yellow pullover shirt, and a red baseball cap that was spattered with white paint and read "Wisconsin" across its front. He looked like a man determined to take it easy.

In truth, however, it was a kind of busman's holiday, for even in repose Carpenter brought along his competitive spirit. "When you are on vacation," he told me one time, "relaxing is a different type of work. When you're hunting, *you* want to be the first to say, 'Duck at three o'clock' or 'Duck from the southwest.'" So it was on a Carpenter fishing trip, in which tradition required that the first person to catch a fish collect a dollar from each of his companions. And if someone else began to pull in more than Jim, he began casting out and reeling in with great urgency.

It was now midmorning, several hours since I had surrendered my dollar. The Charles had yielded plenty of bluegills, and Carpenter even caught a bullhead. He would keep a few to skin and throw in the microwave for dinner, but most were released. Now we were seeking crappie and having little luck. We had motored from spot to spot without even a nibble.

Suddenly, I felt a tremendous yank on my line. Excited, I began reeling it in. Unlike the bluegills, whatever I now had was big and fighting hard. Between its efforts and my fishing inexperience, the top of the rod snapped. Carpenter, perhaps because it was his equipment being mangled, peered over his glasses and watched expectantly. Finally, the creature neared the surface. I muscled it up into the open air.

That was when Jim Carpenter screamed. To hear the man, you would have thought a bullet-riddled victim of the Mob had bubbled to the surface. "That's no fish! That's an eel! It's an eel! Get it out of here! Get it away from the boat! For God's sake, cut it loose!"

Technically, Carp was wrong; an eel is a fish. This one was three feet long, brown and yellow, and squirming insanely.

Jim hurriedly handed me some scissors, again admonishing me to cut the bastard loose. Only after the eel splashed down and twisted away, along with hook and six inches of line, did Carpenter breathe normal again. "I've never liked eels," he said, shuddering. "I caught one one time, and do you know that that thing *smelled* to high heaven? And it was so slippery! Ugh, I hate them."

Carpenter's distaste went back to his boyhood on the farm in Wisconsin. Once when he was about seven, Jim came across what he thought was a deadly water moccasin and crushed the poisonous snake with rocks. He assumed he killed it, but when he looked a bit later, its tail was still moving. More unsettling was the next day, when he returned and the snake was mysteriously gone. Since then Carpenter distrusted snakes and anything resembling them.

The morning drifted on. A gentle rain fell. Our conversation ping-ponged from subject to subject. Carpenter mused about a student in veterinary school who passed out during a lecture, and how when Jim went to help him, the instructor barked, "Leave him be! This always happens around lunchtime."

He also recollected sitting in on some classes at Harvard Medical School and learning that the skeleton in the front of the room was one of the school's former professors.

At one point he called my attention to a mansion on a hill overlooking the river. "That's the house *I'm* going to buy!" he said, sounding like a boy in back of the family station wagon. "And when you come to visit, you can stay down there." He pointed to a cottage that no doubt would come with his purchase.

We settled on the subject of homes, debating whether it was better to buy an existing structure or to build one. Then a funny thought crossed my mind: "Would you ever buy a house if someone had been murdered in it?"

"Sure!" Carpenter said without hesitation. "Especially if it's a good deal. Hell! That wouldn't bother me at all—not at all."

"Wouldn't you be afraid of evil spirits? Or something?"

He shrugged. "I would guess that whoever did the killing would be gone by then, right? That's the only thing I'd be worried about."

We floated some more, quietly. Carpenter considered his lifeless fishing line, then looked over to me. "Now, if it was a house with an eel in it, that would be a different story."

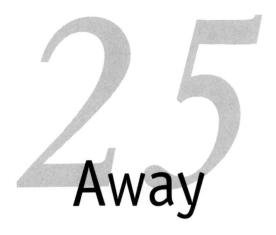

Away

WITH THE ARRIVAL OF AUTUMN, LYNNE MORRIS found herself far from Angell, in North Carolina. Along with her fellow interns, Morris had completed her internship that summer. At the pre-graduation dinner, during which the veterinary staff traditionally lampooned the departing interns, Doug Brum presented her with the Party Animal Award. Like most of the humor that night, it was an inside joke, a reference to Morris's weak stomach at the annual intern party, an occasion she would have preferred to forget. The award was a bottle of tequila, with the worm.

Two weeks after graduation, Morris was married. She and Eric moved directly to Surf City, North Carolina, near Camp LeJeune, where he was stationed as a general medical officer. Another move was scheduled for the following year, to San Diego.

Unlike her fellow interns, who had gone on to residencies and jobs in private practices, Morris now took life easy. Few veterinary jobs were available for someone who would be around only a year. Also, Eric's schedule was such that they could spend plenty of time together—windsurfing, for example, or horseback riding. They adopted a cat. True medical professionals, they named it Horner, after Horner's syndrome, a droopy-eyelid ailment from which the cat suffered.

While Eric was working, Lynne spent a lot of time down on the beach with her dogs, Leah and Graham, walking, playing ball, and thinking. Angell Memorial Animal Hospital was a long way up the coast. Still, it tugged at her. She actually missed those long, intense hours. It made sense why a Doug Brum, who could have doubled his salary in a peaceful private practice, had stayed: It was like being a soldier who endured one harrowing tour of duty, then longed for the battlefield once he got home. Everyday experience paled in comparison. Though unlikely to become reality, given Eric's commitments, Morris also dreamed about returning to Angell, maybe as a resident in medicine.

Rural North Carolina, meanwhile, offered little satisfaction as far as veterinary medicine was concerned. Most of the clinics, Lynne found, were small and outfitted with only basic equipment. For anything but routine care, an owner had to take a pet to the University of North Carolina's veterinary school in Raleigh, three hours away. If pet owners lived in the western part of the state, their best bet was the University of Tennessee, in Knoxville, a seven-hour haul.

Still, Morris wound up helping occasionally at the base veterinary facility and filling in at a nearby clinic. At the clinic the staff was nice enough, but the facilities were lacking. The X ray machine, for instance, was designed for horses. Other basic equipment used by veterinarians all the time was in short supply.

One day Lynne was caring for a dog that had recently undergone surgery for an infected uterus. Now the animal had not urinated for several days. It turned out to be in kidney failure. Anemic, the dog could not even stand. When Lynne went to put the dog on intravenous fluids, she found that none were available. "I couldn't believe it," she said a few days later. "I was there in shock. Immediately, I got on the phone with the owner and said, 'Your dog is dying. You need to take her to a referral hospital, where they can watch her and give her fluids.'

"The bottom line is that the woman wanted to take her and the husband didn't, so they didn't. Now that dog's hanging on, and she may get better or she may not."

In many ways Lynne felt like she was in another world, not only compared to Angell but to most veterinary practices in metropolitan and suburban areas. On the other hand, she was not alone in her dissatisfaction with what she found in the job market. Many veterinary school graduates—and former Angell interns—were disappointed when they went to work, for a salary in the low thirties, and discovered that much of their time was spent with vaccinations and offering advice about treatment for fleas. In many cases the profession failed to live up to expectations. Few owners were willing to spend great amounts on their pets' health. Not many private practices had the wherewithal to perform heroics.

Morris found it difficult, too, to accept that her employer, like many private practitioners, cropped dogs' ears, a procedure that was banned at Angell. That autumn a couple came in with a friendly pit bull terrier puppy. The owner, a Marine, asked that the dog's ears be cut short, because he felt they looked better that way. After surgery, though, the dog's ears remained taped for weeks because they refused to stand upright, as is the fashion.

One day the wife came in and complained about the ears to Lynne. "Look," Morris said, having heard enough, "this dog was *meant* to have floppy ears; they're not supposed to stand up. Just because you surgically do this, doesn't mean they're going to stand."

"Well," said the woman, "what are we going to do if they won't stand?"

"You'll have to ask the person who did the surgery," Morris said, irritated, "because I think it's cruel."

For most of the year, Lynne tried to look to the future. San Diego, she knew, had a number of top-notch practices. As for now, she would make the best of what she could get, even if for the most part, the local vets were only looking for a warm body to help out, not necessarily someone with any special training.

One would-be employer, in fact, glanced at her resume and

noticed that Lynne had done her internship at Angell. "Angell Memorial," he said. "Does this mean you're smarter than me?"

Lynne shook her head. "No," she replied. "It just means that I saw a lot of cases and didn't get any sleep."

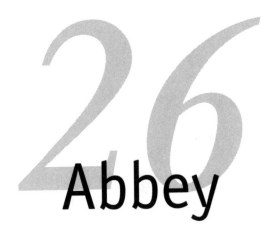

Abbey

IT IS ONE THING TO HAVE OBSERVED STRANGERS AND their animals as they proceeded through Angell's machinery. Day in and day out, people betrayed their true selves through their concern and affection for their pets. Once, I saw a hefty man, who looked like he hauled iron beams for a living, cradle his cat, Poopsie, with the loving gentleness of a first-time mother. I witnessed a woman insanely wailing that her poor dog was bitten on his "pickle" during a skirmish with an adversary. Another time I watched as a professional woman bolted into a back room when she heard her cat shriek at having its surgical staples removed. "Oh, Brave-kins!" she yelled.

After a while I felt a strange brotherhood with Jim Carpenter, for it is very safe to look at the world through a microscope and not have to share anyone's pain.

Things are quite different, however, when it is no longer "they" but you who has the ailing pet.

I got my dog on an autumn afternoon in 1989 and she has been my constant companion ever since. For years I had dreamed about getting a dog, toying with possible breeds and names. As a freelance writer, I worked at home and could make time for a puppy.

Always waiting for the right moment, one day I decided to stop delaying and just do it. I got permission from my landlord, scanned a few books about choosing a dog, made inquiries with a breeder or two, and finally decided that I would get a golden retriever. They were high on the affection scale, low on the bark-o-meter, and size enough to at least be mistaken as protection.

Around that time I saw a classified advertisement for goldens, called, and drove an hour out to St. Mary's Monastery in Petersham, Massachusetts. There I met Brother Andre Bergeron, a bald, whiskered monk of about forty-five years, cloaked in a black robe. He took me around back to an outdoor kennel, where his dog Molly had given birth to a litter of pups, all a rich reddish brown, eight weeks earlier.

There is a reason that advertisers employ golden retriever pup-pies in their commercials: they steal your heart. If selecting a vacuum cleaner is not chore enough, try picking one of eleven yipping balls of fur that will be part of your life for the next ten to fifteen years.

I tried, squatting among those maniacs, and could not. Then I remembered a friend who told me she chose her dog by letting it pick her. In other words, the one that sprang from the litter and paid her the most attention was the one she took home. It is a ridiculous strategy if you think about it. In essence, you are basing a longtime commitment on the indiscernible whim of a puppy.

All I really knew was that I preferred a female, mainly because my family had good luck with female dogs when I was growing up. So I asked Brother Andre to place the three females about five feet in front of me and announced that the one to come forward would be forever mine.

Brother Andre rounded up the pups. Slowly, he stooped low and set them on the ground before me. It was the moment of truth. Each of them then looked and considered me for a wide-eyed instant. Then they all turned and ran.

A friend would later joke that I took the one that fled slowest. The truth was that I finally selected a pup based on a distinguishing tuft of white hair on her chest. Born at a monastery, she became Abbey.

The canine universe is divided into dominant and submissive dogs, all in varying degrees, with each possessing an innate ability to sort it all out. Abbey, I would soon learn, got along by deferring. Though she had rare flashes of ferocity, she usually dealt with new dogs and intimidating people by hugging the earth. If particularly excited, she would simply roll over and urinate. Not the noblest position, but in dog circles it did the trick.

Having a dog was natural to me. My family had owned two poodles when I was young. But even when we didn't have one, neighborhood dogs were ever-present. I also like to walk. Taking Abbey out—at any hour, in any weather—was undaunting. If anything, she provided an explanation for why I was slogging through a downpour or a blizzard.

Furthermore, she was the intermediary in meeting hundreds of people. One day I was sitting on a bench on the campus of Boston College, up the street from my apartment. I was reading a paperback, and Abbey was perched next to me, taking in the passersby, when an older gentleman—a professor, was my guess—stepped over. He seemed downcast but brightened as he stroked her fur. She leaned against him, basking in the attention. "Ah," the man said mournfully, "if only people were like golden retrievers."

At least in temperament. Unfortunately, indiscriminate breeding has resulted in innumerable golden retrievers with a propensity for hip dysplasia, certain cancers, and other ailments. By age three Abbey remained in good health—knock on wood.

I had kept my Angell veterinarian, Jean Duddy, during the course of this book and hoped the day would never come that I had to count on the hospital for much more than vaccinations and heartworm pills. At three in the morning on Thanksgiving, however, the retching started. I was asleep when I heard the telltale whining and opened my eyes to see her staring me in the face, looking distressed and in search of comforting. I hurried to get some newspapers, and sure enough, up came dinner.

A fact of life is that dogs do vomit periodically. Outdoors, even on a leash, they find ways to eat the most unappetizing things, with grass being the least revolting. While they regurgitate less often than cats, it is with equal gusto and apparent pleasure.

You start to worry, though, when it continues. Neither of us got much sleep that night, as the vomiting carried on almost every hour on the hour. On into Thanksgiving it went, through dinner and televised football, until she had nothing left to cough up. When I took her out, diarrhea was the order of the day.

I, meanwhile, was almost keeling over with fatigue and bewilderment. Even when I dozed off for fifteen minutes or so, part of me was still awake, listening for her next attack. Parents with infants, I imagine, essentially face the same problem: something is obviously wrong, but communication is impossible. I searched my memory and looked around for signs of missing foodstuffs, tampered-with rubbish, damaged belongings. Nothing seemed amiss.

By afternoon the dog was sagging, her eyes sunken, her tail tucked between her legs, and she rejected food and water. Finally—later than I probably should have—I packed her in the car and drove the few miles to Jamaica Plain. Intern Beth Shurland was holding down Fort Angell when I arrived about seven o'clock. The place was almost empty, though I had been told that Thanksgiving and the day after could get busy with pets sick from too much human food and the ever-present threat of turkey bones.

Shurland smiled a little, I thought, when she saw my dog and me sitting there, looking forlorn. "What are *you* doing here?" she said brightly.

"Beth there's no place I would rather not be."

"Me, too," she said, grinning.

About average height, Shurland wore a short, professional hairstyle and held herself with a calm not always found in interns. Indeed, she was not among those regularly summoned to Paul Gambardella's office to explain or counter the arguments of one angry client or another. A little older than the typical intern, she tended to keep control of situations with owners. And when it came down to it, she seemed comfortable admitting if she simply didn't know an answer.

Now just a few weeks shy of twenty-nine years old, Beth came to veterinary medicine in a roundabout way. She had wanted to be a vet since she was six. As an undergraduate at Tufts, however, she was disillusioned by the cutthroat competition in the sciences and abandoned her dream. She took most of the prerequisites for veterinary school, but instead of biology she majored in English literature. After graduating in 1985, Shurland took a job with a publisher, hawking textbooks up and down the northeast seaboard for the better part of two years. It was lonely and unsatisfying. She hated it.

In despair one night, she turned to her husband, Abe, and asked just what was she going to do with her life. He shrugged. "Why don't you go to vet school?" he suggested. The cartoon-style lightbulb blinked on over Beth's head.

One thing led to another. She took a position as an attendant at Angell to get some experience. Then she entered veterinary school at Tufts. Now, after graduating in June, she found herself an intern at the same place that her family brought their pets when she was growing up in the Boston suburb of Reading.

As always, Beth adored the animals. She was also discovering that a lot of the people were OK, too. Unexpectedly, one client asked her to be her pet's full-time veterinarian. Another one came in with a gift of a Megabucks lottery ticket—"So you can open your own clinic." "So far, so good" was Beth's summation of her new profession.

Shurland ushered us into an examination room. Scanning Abbey's file, she listened to my story. She asked whether Abbey had perhaps eaten something, whether a toy or anything else small and ingestible was missing. It was a routine question, given that Abbey was a young golden retriever. ("Do you want a brain with that model?" was Joan Fontaine's standard commentary on the breed.)

Like all the interns, Shurland had seen her share of foreign bodies in her five months at Angell. She had one cat who died after it ate string, which then got hung up, pulled taut, and sawed open its innards—gruesome, but not particularly uncommon. Another cat had eaten a tiny spring, which pierced the intestine wall and started winding its way out. One dog had a piece of tennis ball lodged in its gut. And just a week or two before Abbey's arrival, Beth was visited by an

Airedale with a perfume bottle in its gastrointestinal tract. Experience was probably behind her unconvinced "Uh-huh," when I said that Abbey never ate anything but perishables.

Beth inspected my dog up and down. She pulled back her jowl and found her gums still pink. A couple times, she lifted the loose skin on Abbey's back, then dropped it to see whether her skin was still elastic, another test for dehydration.

Next she ran her fingers along Abbey's abdomen, pressing here, squeezing there, until she lingered around the middle. "It feels like there could be a tubular mass right here," she said, fingering a loop of intestine.

"Tubular mass" could mean a lot of things. Beth's biggest worry was an intussusception. In other words, it was possible that the intestine was for some reason telescoping in on itself. If that were the case, emergency surgery would be needed. It was true that an intussusception sometimes will correct itself, but if it doesn't, it can cut off the flow of blood and begin killing tissue and, in the end, the animal.

But it was a difficult call to make. Sometimes what seemed like thickened intestine upon palpation was in reality a stool. And while you didn't want to cut a dog open needlessly, waiting too long could be fatal.

Oddly enough, I had recently been on the telephone with Lynne Morris in North Carolina, and she recounted a similar experience, one of her worst at Angell. It was a boxer named Duke, and between money problems and Lynne's inability to reach the owner on the phone, surgery was delayed six long hours. When the surgeon finally opened Duke up, he found the havoc caused by an intussusception—nine feet of blackened, rotting intestine. Still, the animal survived.

"Abbey," Shurland said, "I see an X ray in your future." We brought her down to radiology—the dog resisting every step of the process—but the radiographs only confused matters. Being a one-dimensional view of a three-dimensional animal, a radiograph of a dog's innards can be tricky to interpret. Certain sections end up layered upon one another, making it difficult to sort everything out.

Large intestine, in particular, can be mistaken for small intestine dangerously enlarged with backed-up gas. Though no definite foreign body could be seen in Abbey's case, it did not mean that something undetectable, like a sock or countless other items, wasn't there.

Beth mulled it over. Rather than call in a surgeon that night, she thought we could wait until morning to see how Abbey felt, then let Jean Duddy look her over as well. Abbey was lethargic; the initial bloodwork suggested some dehydration; but she was not in immediate danger. I agreed that waiting was best.

Abbey would be admitted, put on intravenous fluids for the night, and monitored by the nurses in ICU. As with people, dehydration was to be taken seriously. After so much vomiting, an animal's electrolyte balance can be severely thrown out of whack. And if a dog or cat is flirting with another illness, such as kidney disease or diabetes, dehydration can spark a crisis.

Beth filled out some paperwork and threw a hospital leash around my dog's neck. I walked out carrying an empty collar and leash.

Sleep came slowly that evening. I was worried, true, but there was also a silence that blanketed my room. I imagine city dwellers who spend a night in the peaceful country must suffer a similar void. It wasn't the hum of traffic that I longed for, of course, but the gentle rhythm of a dog's sleeping breath.

ON ROUNDS THE NEXT MORNING, JEAN DUDDY, Shurland, and three or four other interns went through the paces of discussing what animals came in overnight and their treatment plans. When they got to my dog, they brought her out of her cage and, as they do with most animals, gathered around to have a look. Ever friendly but ever wary, Abbey dropped to her back and proceeded to sprinkle half of the veterinarians with urine. Then, slapping her tail in the puddle, she managed to splash the rest. (Duddy—a 31-year-old earth-mother type—would later reprimand me with a smile and a wag of the finger: "You didn't warn us that she was a submissive pee-er.")

The indications were that Abbey was improving. IV fluids were helping her dehydration. She had not vomited since the early morning hours. She seemed to have fluid-filled intestines, but they were causing no pain.

The plan was to take another round of X rays and see what they showed. As likely as not, it could very well just have been a virus or an upset stomach from something she ate. Most likely, if the dog continued to not vomit, she could have water that night and probably go home the next day, Saturday.

It was when the second set of radiographs came back that the confusion started. Strangely, the X ray technician had managed to capture the intestines in the midst of identical contractions in films that were taken ten minutes apart. This was a fluke, but by itself the coincidence might suggest not contractions but an obstruction.

Then, as Shurland inspected the films and explained her uncertainty to a colleague, a passing surgeon happened to take a peek. "If that was my dog," the woman said without hesitation, "I would cut it." Interns at Angell make their own choices. But if a permanent staff member makes such a pronouncement, doubts creep in—or, in some instances, cascade in.

Shurland got a hold of Duddy. Now Jean went back and scanned the X rays herself. She, too, was uncertain whether the films revealed an enlarged small colon or a normal large colon. What she knew for certain, though, was that the dog herself seemed to be doing OK. "You always need to look at the animal," Duddy told me later. "You can look at an X ray of a dog that has a severe pneumothorax after being hit by a car. If you looked at the X ray, you might think, 'Man, this dog must be gasping for air,' but in reality the dog is sitting in ICU like it doesn't have a care in the world. On X rays alone, you might say, 'God, this dog needs a chest tube,' but then when you look at the dog, you think, 'Hmmmm—do we do anything, or do we just wait it out and let the body heal itself?'

"It's the same with blood work. You can look at a piece of paper that says an animal's kidney values are four times normal and say, 'Oh, God—this animal's dying.' Well, if you don't know the animal, you don't know the situation. This may have been going on for six months, and this dog or cat is still running around looking perfectly normal. It happens all the time.

"One thing that I repeat over and over to my clients is that I will not treat pieces of paper. I had a client in yesterday who says that if her cat's suffering, she's going to put it to sleep. And this cat looks perfectly normal. Well, we rechecked its kidney values and they're three times normal. I told her, 'Well, your cat still looks normal. If you want to put the piece of paper to sleep, I'll be glad to.'"

When I showed up around eleven-thirty that morning, Duddy gave me some options. A surgeon could cut Abbey open, she said, and look around for the obstruction. But, if I wanted, we could probably hold off until the radiologist, who had been off for the holiday, was available and get a more expert evaluation of the X rays.

Surgery was the safest route. Still, I had been around the dog all day when she first fell sick. I could think of nothing—not a Q-tip nor a Ring Ding wrapper nor a corncob—that she might have eaten. What's more, I didn't think she *would* eat them. Without reason, I dismissed the possibility of an intussusception. It did not help that I was so low on money that I had gone to a longtime friend for help in paying this ever-growing bill.

I asked Duddy about the risks. She said nothing was certain, but it seemed safe to wait. Abbey was in stable condition. "The real dilemma," Duddy would tell me, "comes when you know there's an obstruction, and it's three in the morning, and you think, 'God, should we wait until morning and cut the dog then, or should we do it now?' At this place, we tend to call in the surgeon and cut it."

Certainly that was the philosophy that Shurland brought with her from Tufts. "The thing they told us in school, and I think it's true, is that it's better to cut a dog that doesn't need to be cut than not to cut a dog that should be cut," she told me later. "Doing an abdominal exploratory is *not* that big a deal. It sounds like it to the owner, but if you see them doing them, and if you see enough of them, you realize it's just not that big a deal.

"In clinics at school one time, a surgeon was on, and three possible foreign bodies came in. She took the first one into surgery, and it was negative—no foreign body—nothing. She took the second one—nothing. So she didn't take the third one—"

I figured even I could finish this story: "And *that* one had a foreign body."

"No," Beth said, giving me a look. "That one would have been negative, too. The point is that the X rays were equivocal. Maybe the animal was obstructed; maybe not.

"With Abbey, it would have been reasonable to take her to surgery, and it was reasonable not to. That's why it was important to have you involved. Some people would say 'Cut her, definitely,' and some people are more conservative. You have to kind of work that into it, too."

Back in the midst of the crisis, I then told Jean Duddy I would rather wait for the radiologist's opinion. Jean seemed to intimate that this was her inclination as well.

Feeling a little gloomy—over Abbey's health, over a decision that was based more on hope than anything else, and over a mounting bill—I poked my head into an office where Doug Brum was making some calls. "It sucks" was Brum's summary of my situation. Over the past year, I had heard Doug use that phrase a thousand times. Dog died? It sucks. Lost your job? It sucks. If a mighty tornado were someday to drive Boston to its knees, I felt confident that I could predict Brum's exact words as he stepped through the ruins. At the moment, however, he struck me as remarkably sage for such a young man.

He also told me to fear not. "Garbage," he said. "I'll bet you anything that dog just got into the garbage."

Later that day radiologist Lori Hartzband slid Abbey's films up on her light screen and ran her eyes over them for a minute or two. "There's no obstruction," she said matter-of-factly. "What's next?" her body language said as she distractedly scanned a row of films from another sick pet.

Next on my list was to take Abbey home. They kept her one more night—until she ate some solid food—scrawled "gastroenteritis" in her file, and handed me a bill for $421.47.

I settled the paperwork. Then, feeling my oats, I sneaked Abbey down a hall where animals were prohibited, to say good-bye to Jean Duddy and some of the liaisons. They came over to pat her, huddling around. Merrily, I thought, my beautiful russet dog flopped onto her back and let loose a geyser.

Epilogue

AFTER A YEAR OF TREADING WATER IN NORTH Carolina, Lynne Morris and husband Eric Smith moved to San Diego in the summer of 1993. On August 21 that year, Lynne gave birth to her first child, Travis Morris Smith, who weighed in at seven pounds twelve ounces.

Eric spent two years at a naval hospital there, fulfilling his residency requirements. In April 1994, meanwhile, Lynne found a job as a staff veterinarian at the Emergency Animal Hospital in San Diego. It was a four-doctor practice that, as its named suggested, handled only emergencies, perfect for Morris. She worked thirteen-hour shifts, usually at night, once or twice during the week and every other weekend.

In many ways Morris had found an ideal job. She missed seeing the relatively healthy animals that are the mainstays of most veterinary practices: vaccinations, checkups, fleas. At the same time, she was spared the balloon-bursting ennui that many young veterinarians experience upon entering the workaday world. For Morris every new patient was an adventure.

And to some degree a case of déjà vu. "You know what it's like?" she asked me. "It's like doing overnights at Angell. That's all I do: overnights. It's not uncommon for me to get three hit-by-cars coming in the door in a ten-minute period. You just need to say, 'OK, that one's pink; this one is dying—we need to get approval for a catheter and fluids; and this one's, well, whatever. It's not always like that, but it is exciting and much more fun than most jobs."

She started grinding her teeth as she slept, however, so perhaps work was more stressful, as well.

Like her experience at Angell, Morris was gathering plenty of stories about colorful clients. Her favorite was the woman who showed up with her hairless little yip-yip dog, owner and pet wearing matching green silk jackets. The "emergency" that brought them to Lynne was a pimple on Fifi's belly. When that problem was resolved, Morris remembered, the woman proceeded to produce from her pocketbook a little white rabbit in a harness, a newly purchased accessory for her canine companion. "What do you think of *this?*" she asked proudly.

There was bad news, too. At Christmas I received a card from Lynne mentioning that one of her two dogs, Leah, had died of a ruptured splenic tumor. "Other than having broken hearts," she wrote, "we are well."

Lynne worked at the San Diego hospital a little more than a year. In the summer of 1995, Eric's military commitments called again, and this time the family was off for Spain, where Eric would complete his internal medicine residency at a military installation south of Seville. Lynne went to work at a low-level veterinary clinic on the base and focused on learning Spanish, sight-seeing, and having another child, due in July 1996.

Paul Gambardella, for his part, never quite resolved the tug-of-war between his love for surgery and the administrative demands of his job as chief of staff. When I revisited him late in 1995, in fact, he had taken on additional duties, a three-year stint as president of the American College of Veterinary Surgeons, that kept him out of the O.R. even more.

Burdens remained. The satellite operation in Lexington proved to be a debacle and closed after a short time. In December 1995 former veterinarian Marjorie McMillan was awarded $787,000 in back pay and punitive damages in her sex discrimination lawsuit against the hospital, stunning the chief of staff.

Still, when I saw him, Gambardella seemed more content in his job. The hospital was about to begin kidney transplants for cats and add a $1 million radiation therapy section. There had also been some high-level veterinary staff changes, among them the retirement of his sometime nemesis, pathologist Jim Carpenter. There were a good number of new veterinarians around the place and fewer long-timers. I got the feeling that this was finally becoming Gambardella's own staff, not just one he inherited.

Patient visits at the Boston hospital were up again, hovering around forty-four thousand, and the budget was largely under control. Once he spoke of laying off a veterinarian or two, but now Gambardella was talking about adding staff, including a second veterinarian in ICU. If it happened, that would be a big change for the interns. Two ICU veterinarians would mean that the critical-care ward would be manned by experienced staff more hours each week. In short, the new doctors would have more help during those fearsome late-night shifts.

I found Jim Carpenter in his native Wisconsin. In June 1994 he had retired from Angell after 33 years. He accepted a deep cut in pay to accept a job working as a staff pathologist for a friend and former colleague at a busy clinic in Marshfield, around the center of the state.

He was still working ten-to-twelve-hour days, but now only four times a week. His wife, Grace, had fallen seriously ill and, happily, recovered. Carpenter saw death every day in his work, but it took the near-loss of a loved one to make it hit home that life was short.

These days Carp took more time with Grace and found plenty of occasions to enjoy the outdoors with his brother Doug. Jim bought what he described as a "big-boy toy," an all-terrain vehicle, which he enjoyed immensely.

Carpenter also learned to bowhunt since I had seen him last. He had even claimed his first deer without a gun, admitting that it was unsettling to hear the awful sound of an arrow striking bone when he failed to hit the animal chest-center.

It didn't sound like he longed for much about Angell Memorial Animal Hospital, until I reminded him of the huge collection of case slides dating back to the 1940s. The pathologist had used those samples for countless papers and teaching his residents. He sighed and admitted that he wished he could put his hands on those to help make his points when speaking with some of his fellow pathologists. "You bet I miss that," he said.

Doug Brum, meanwhile, continued to speed through Angell's halls, being a balm to sick pets, their owners, and everyone else who needed a listening ear or a pat on the back.

Toward the end of my stay, Doug and his wife went on a month-long hiking trip in the western states. They trekked through a variety of national parks, from Olympic in Washington to Grand Canyon in Arizona, and thought they had escaped Angell's mighty pull. That is, until one day on a lonely trail in North Cascades National Park, when from out of the blue appeared a former Angell medicine resident and her family. (Brum shouldn't have been too surprised: author Peter Jenkins, of *A Walk Across America* fame, wrote about meeting a onetime Angell intern while doing the legwork for *Across China*.)

Doug and Sue had two sons since I had left the hospital—Benjamin, who was born June 24, 1993, and Jared, who came June 4, 1995. Benjamin's first movie was *Free Willy*, which, knowing Brum, somehow didn't surprise me.

And though Doug took a month or two off after each of the births, it did not take long for him to return to the maelstrom. His friends at the hospital confided that he was more stressed than ever. He had surrendered his job as director of the interns, but even that did not help much. "No matter how busy I was before," Doug admitted, "I'm a lot more busy now."

Intensive care nurse Joan Fontaine had been active as well. In December 1995 she testified against the hospital in the gender-based discrimination lawsuit brought by former veterinarian Marjorie McMillan, which surely won her no friends in management. (Yet it was Fontaine—and no one else—who called me, with a certain excitement, to report that Angell was highlighted in the latest issue of *Yankee* magazine and that the hospital had again appeared on "Rescue 911.")

Joan remained at Angell. She had thrown herself into moving on to a career in human health care. Undaunted by rejections for medical school, she signed up for even more academic courses, volunteered as an emergency room aide at Boston's Brigham and

Women's Hospital, and launched a new series of college applications, this time for physician assistant programs.

With a few more years of schooling in her future, Fontaine was delaying getting another dog. I got the feeling, too, that she missed the one she had lost. A few months after Duke died, in fact, Fontaine paid fifty dollars to the International Star Registry in Switzerland to have one of the infinite number of luminaries named after him. Duke's star is in the Constellation Lynx between Ursa Major and Gemini. "The coordinates are RQ, 8H, 24M, 25SD, 34 degrees, 34 minutes," she told me. "And the name of that star is Duke Caribou Fontaine."

The more I thought about that, the more I liked it. Perhaps all of our creatures deserve as much: to hold forever a place in the heavens, bright lights all.